The Medical Follow-up Agency

THE FIRST FIFTY YEARS
1946–1996

Edward D. Berkowitz and Mark J. Santangelo

NATIONAL ACADEMY PRESS
Washington, D.C.

NATIONAL ACADEMY PRESS • **2101 Constitution Avenue, NW** • **Washington, DC 20418**

Additional copies of *The Medical Follow-up Agency: The First Fifty Years, 1946–1996*, are available for sale from the National Academy Press, Box 285, 2101 Constitution Avenue, N.W., Washington, DC 20055. Call (800) 624-6242 or (202) 334-3313 (in the Washington metropolitan area), or visit the National Academy Press's on-line bookstore at *www.nap.edu*.

For more information about the Medical Follow-up Agency, visit the MFUA home page at *www2.nas.edu/mfua*.

International Standard Book No. 0-309-06440-6

Cover: Marines on conditioning march, summer 1997; the School of Infantry, Camp Geiger, North Carolina. Original photo courtesy of Mathew Lynch.

Preface

During World War II, the 15 million servicemen mobilized and deployed around the world produced an extraordinarily large and complex medical experience. The medical care provided by the armed forces was thorough and competent. A consultant system of leading medical scientists in all clinical disciplines was deployed and assigned to major commands in all zones of operation, both in the United States and overseas. Many distinguished medical teaching centers established affiliated general hospital units with research-minded faculty personnel, who were assigned to, and saw active service in, all overseas theaters of operation. Medical observations and data were recorded and centrally indexed. Medical problems in virtually all clinical disciplines, including trauma, surgery, infectious diseases, and psychiatry, often assumed urgent military importance and accordingly generated research and innovative therapeutic measures. Affiliated research activities of military import were also being provided by various committees of the National Research Council of the National Academy of Sciences.

Toward the end of the war, it became increasingly apparent that a vast amount of medical data and research observations on a wide array of medical problems had been accumulated, strongly suggesting the opportunity for follow-up studies. Accordingly, on March 5, 1946, I submitted a memorandum to Surgeon General Norman Kirk, pointing out that "an enormous amount of material of great clinical value" had accumulated in the medical records kept by the armed services, such that, in fact, "[i]t can fairly be said that no similar amount of material has ever been accumulated, and it is doubtful whether a similar amount will ever again be available." I then proposed to turn this material to a "practical use by the establishment of a clinical research program, including a follow-up system to determine the natural and post-treatment history of such diseases and conditions as might be selected for the study." By this means, it would be possible to ascertain the long-term effects of various forms of treatment, as well as the natural history of certain pathologic processes. I further stated that "[t]hese and other data, departing from a given base line and followed-up over long periods of time dispassionately and in the absence of special pleading, have never been available."

I proposed that the project be a joint undertaking of the Army and the Veterans Administration, with the National Research Council assuming an important role in appointing a committee to initiate and implement the project and to "exercise a general supervisory function." I suggested that funding might be obtained through a direct federal subsidy or through a National Research Foundation, for which legislation was then pending and which later evolved into the National Science Foundation.

Fortunately, Surgeon General Kirk heartily accepted my memorandum and recommended its consideration to the National Academy of Sciences–National Research Council. The enthusiastic and expeditious response of the Academy and the committees it established to assess the proposal and "explore the most effective means by which a medical research program utilizing this material can be carried out" is reflected in the fact that by May 7, 1946, less than two months after I wrote my memorandum to Surgeon General Kirk, a Committee on Veteran Medical Problems was appointed under the chairmanship of Dr. Edward D. Churchill. The committee directed the staff, which was then composed of Dr. Gilbert W. Beebe and me (we were both still in the military and assigned by the surgeon general to the National Academy of Sciences–National Research Council on temporary duty to work on this project) "to prepare the groundwork for Committee action."

Dr. Beebe and I therefore prepared a "draft report of the character and scope of the follow-up proposal and the mission, structure, organization, and funding support." This report was discussed and generally approved by the committee at its final meeting on June 13, 1946. Within only about three months of my original proposal, on March 5, 1946, the program thus became operational under the aegis of the National Research Council, with the appointment of Dr. Beebe as its first full-time statistical analyst.

As the originator of this program, I am most gratified to observe the impressive medical scientific contributions emanating from its activities during its half century of existence, as well as the valuable tangential contributions made in setting the standards for the procedures and mechanisms of follow-up studies. These standards have greatly influenced subsequent studies, such as epidemiologic investigations, multicenter controlled clinical trials, and so-called outcomes research. In great measure this has been due to the capable leadership of Gilbert Beebe, followed by that of Seymour Jablon, and more recently, Richard N. Miller, along with the dedicated advisory support of a wide array of scientists.

As may be readily evident from this historical document, I am pleased that the original purpose of this program, both in vision and in reality, has been fully achieved. It has, however, "been considerably amplified, both in terms of its immediate advancement in medical scientific knowledge and in its impact on future endeavors in this field," as exemplified by the expansive and vigorous medical research activities of the armed forces and the Veterans Administration, which were virtually nonexistent before World War II.

Michael E. DeBakey, M.D.
Olga Keith Weiss and Distinguished
Service Professor of Surgery, and
Director, DeBakey Heart Center

Foreword

The Medical Follow-up Agency is a national treasure for veterans and for long-term studies of health. Its data resources provide incomparable opportunities to follow very important populations and to ask creative questions about their well-being as well as the occurrence and significance of illness. The Twin Registry provides an opportunity to understand the impact of heredity on health and disease in a population of more than 16,000 pairs of twins (i.e., 32,000 veterans).

The Medical Follow-up Agency is a living tribute to the vision, energy, and effectiveness of Michael E. DeBakey, M.D. Dr. DeBakey created the idea for the agency, obtained the appropriate approvals, staffed its initial creation, and 50 years later, spoke on the occasion of its golden anniversary. This sequence of events must be unique in the history of veterans' health and medical research.

I congratulate the staff and the volunteers who have made the Medical Follow-up Agency so useful and effective over the past 50 years. This history is a testimony to their contributions. Support by the Departments on Defense and Veterans Affairs, and by the National Institutes of Health, has been crucial to the success of the agency. It is my hope that the partnership of staff, volunteers, scientists, and these government agencies will continue to provide useful information for health well into the next millennium.

Kenneth I. Shine, M.D.
President, Institute of Medicine

Authors' Acknowledgments

The authors of this monograph would like to thank the staff of the Medical Follow-up Agency (MFUA) and of the National Academy of Sciences archives for their considerable help. We are also grateful to the people who took the time to sit for formal oral interviews about the founding and development of the MFUA, namely, Dr. Gilbert Beebe, Dr. Michael DeBakey, Mr. Seymour Jablon, Dr. Richard Miller, and Dr. William Page.

The authors would also like to acknowledge the contributions of Mr. Seymour Jablon, Dr. Lois Joellenbeck, Dr. Richard Miller, Dr. Robert Miller, Dr. James Norman, and Dr. William Page, who worked to prepare the study summaries located throughout this manuscript. Ms. Heather O'Maonaigh of the MFUA provided invaluable technical and editorial support to the authors during the production of this history.

Finally, we would like to thank the reviewers of the manuscript: Dr. Gilbert Beebe, Mr. Seymour Jablon, Dr. John Kurtzke, Dr. James Norman, and Dr. Eldon Sutton. Thanks are also due to Ms. Florence Poillon, who served as consulting editor for the final draft of this publication.

Edward D. Berkowitz   Mark J. Santangelo

Contents

Boxes

The Medical Follow-up Agency

1

Creating the Agency

Although the Second World War caused mass destruction, it also served as a source of much scientific progress. The field of medicine was one discipline that was able to benefit from this wartime progress. National mobilization led to the provision of medical care on a scale unknown in American history. Not only were many of the nation's young adults pressed into wartime service, so too were its doctors. The nation's leading medical schools assembled units of doctors who treated wartime casualties and provided routine medical care to members of the armed forces. As a result, millions of people who previously had seen a doctor sporadically, if at all, began to receive comprehensive care. These medical encounters produced a large set of medical records that constituted a potential resource for clinicians and statisticians. The Medical Follow-up Agency grew out of a desire to use these records to improve medical care and learn more about the course of disease.

THE IDEA

After the surrender of Japan in August 1945, the nation's attention shifted to the process of demobilization. During the war, the National Academy of Sciences (NAS), acting through the Division of Medical Sciences of its National Research Council, had provided advice to the surgeons general of the Army and Navy on medical research and other matters related to wartime care. Between 1940 and 1946, advisory committees on war services held more than 700 meetings and 243 conferences and played an important role in shaping the nation's wartime medical policy.[1] In 1946, however, the National Research Council (NRC) contemplated an end to these emergency activities. At the beginning of the year, Dr. Lewis H. Weed, the chairman of the Division of Medical Services, reported that all of the committees would be discharged by the end of June. At the same time, negotiations were under way to forge a new relationship with the surgeons general of the Army, Navy, Public Health Service, and Veterans Administration. Weed expected the division "to be intimately concerned with research problems undertaken by the principal federal agencies concerned with medicine."[2]

On March 12, 1946, Major General Norman T. Kirk, the surgeon general of the United States Army, wrote to Frank B. Jewett, the president of the National Academy of Sciences, and suggested that conferences be held to discuss a new advisory relationship between the Academy and the federal medical agencies. Within three weeks, a preliminary conference took place in which the participants agreed that "strong efforts" should be made to continue the services of the National Research Council. An ensuing conference on postwar research held on April 18 at the National Academy of Sciences attracted 43 people, among them some of the nation's leaders in medical administration and medical research. Dr. Edward Churchill, a professor of surgery at the Harvard Medical School, chaired the meeting. Those in attendance included Louis Dublin, who had done pioneering work in health statistics with the Metropolitan Life Insurance Company; William Menninger of the famous psychiatric family; Barnes Woodhall, a distinguished clinician and medical researcher from Duke; and John Whitehorn, the chief of the psychiatry department at Johns Hopkins.[3] Faculty members from the medical schools at Northwestern, Western Reserve, Columbia, Vanderbilt, Pennsylvania, and Yale also attended.

Even in the presence of so much senior medical talent, Colonel Michael E. DeBakey of the Army's Office of the Surgeon General, a surgeon who subsequently came to international fame in his field, played the key role at the meeting. A memo that he had sent to General Kirk on March 5, 1946, served as the basis for the discussion. In this memo, DeBakey pointed out that "an enormous amount of material" had accumulated in the medical records kept by the armed services. "It can fairly be said," he wrote, "that no similar amount of material has ever been accumulated, and it is doubtful whether a similar amount will ever again be available." DeBakey proposed to turn this material to "practical use by the establishment of a clinical research program, including a follow-up system to determine the natural and post-treatment history" of the diseases and conditions treated during the war. DeBakey offered the example of peptic ulcer as a condition that might be studied. A follow-up of cases identified during the war would establish the conditions under which the ulcers led to perforation, hemorrhage, and other complications. Such an exercise could enable clinicians to settle such questions as whether "benign peptic ulcers undergo malignant changes." Investigators would also be able to ascertain the long-term effects of various forms of treatment. "These and other data, departing from a given base line and followed up over long periods of time, dispassionately and in the absence of special pleading,

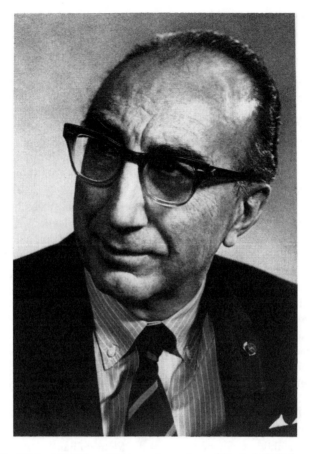

Dr. Michael DeBakey. Photograph courtesy of Dr. Lois DeBakey.

have never been available," DeBakey noted. Among other conditions that might benefit from such an approach were head injuries, bone defects, and peripheral nerve injuries.

In DeBakey's memo lay the origins of the Medical Follow-up Agency. He envisioned the project as a joint undertaking between the Army and the Veterans Administration (VA). He also saw a role for the National Research Council, which would appoint a committee to initiate and implement the project and, in DeBakey's words, "exercise a general supervisory function." This method of operation would continue the successful partnership between the NAS and the federal government that had been established during the war. To finance the enterprise, DeBakey thought funds might be obtained through a National

Research Foundation, should Congress choose to establish one (this notion later evolved into the National Science Foundation), or through a direct federal subsidy.[4]

At the April conference on postwar medical research, DeBakey's idea received a favorable response, both from key government officials and from private practitioners. General Menninger, who, like DeBakey himself, would soon return to civilian practice, pointed to the need for such follow-up activities in psychiatry. He noted that little was known about the long-term effects of such conditions as battle fatigue. Barnes Woodhall mentioned that studies had already begun regarding soldiers who had received operations for peripheral nerve injuries. Others cited the value of the work that could be done in such fields as the treatment of epilepsy and cancer.

Dr. Paul Magnuson, assistant medical director of the Veterans Administration medical program, endorsed the proposal and noted that the VA was prepared to supply funds to carry it out. Dr. Robert Dyer, director of the National Institutes of Health—which were just beginning their period of tremendous postwar growth—became enthusiastic over the chance "to follow a whole generation of men and trace their life history." He called it an "unparalleled" opportunity. Louis Dublin agreed that "there was nothing comparable to this opportunity in the entire world." To miss it would be "utterly tragic." Indeed, a similar discussion had taken place after the First World War, but the opportunity had been lost.[5] Dublin's comments underscored the desire not to repeat the mistakes that had been made after the World War I. Rather than simply return to the status quo ante as it had done then, American medicine would now put to use the clinical experience of the Second World War.

Most of the attendees realized that a new type of relationship between the government and the medical profession would govern medical research in the postwar era. Dublin, a vice-president of the Metropolitan Life Insurance Company, noted that there were projects, such as the one DeBakey was proposing, that were simply beyond the scope of private companies. What his company could do was small compared to what could be done with the military records that, as one doctor noted, covered 10 to 12 percent of the population. Dublin also warned that the work would have to be carried out by "highly skilled personnel" and not by the "ordinary physician." He implied that this effort would require the assistance of statisticians and would fall into the domain of academic medical centers.

Dr. Churchill selected three participants to draft a resolution that would express the sense of the conference. With unanimity and with the Veterans Administration eager to have the National Research Council assume an advisory role in its postwar research program, the group passed the resolution immediately. Urging the nation to seize an "unparalleled opportunity," the group recommended that the NRC appoint a committee "to explore the most effective means by which a medical research program . . . can be carried out, to the end that the care of patients, the investigation of disease, and the improvement of medical practice and education be advanced."[6]

ORGANIZING A PLAN OF ACTION

This first meeting led to another when, on May 7, 1946, a temporary Committee on Veterans' Medical Problems met at the National Academy of Sciences to formulate a plan of action. Once again, Dr. Churchill chaired the meeting. Eight others joined him on the committee, six of whom worked in leading medical centers. Churchill explained the group's mission as preparing a report to the National Research Council that would serve as "a basis for action."[7]

To research and write the report, the committee relied on DeBakey and Gilbert W. Beebe, who had been detailed to the NRC from the Army's Office of the Surgeon General. DeBakey, who had directed the Surgeon General's Surgical Consultants Division, held the civilian job of assistant professor of surgery at

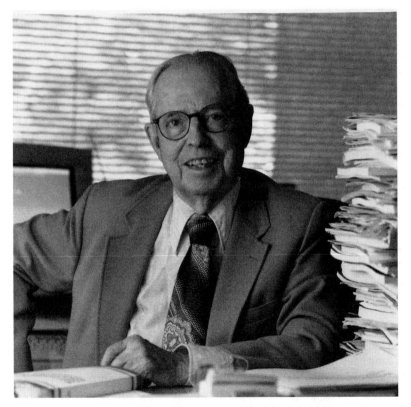

Dr. Gilbert Beebe—1996. Photo by Bill Branson, courtesy of Dr. Gilbert Beebe.

Tulane. A persuasive writer, he brought a clinician's perspective to the task. Beebe, who had headed the Analysis and Reporting Branch of the Control Division in the Surgeon General's Office, held a Ph.D. in sociology and statistics. In civilian life, Beebe had worked at the Milbank Memorial Fund, an important institution in epidemiology and in what a later generation would call health services research.[8]

Much of the discussion centered on the structure of the organization that would perform follow-up work. DeBakey envisioned a committee of prominent physicians volunteering their time in the traditional NAS manner that would select appropriate projects and oversee the agency. An operating body, composed of full-time employees of the National Research Council with expertise in statistics and research design, would complement this directing body. One important task of this body would be to prepare the rosters of individuals to be used in particular studies, using information provided by the Army and the Navy. The studies themselves, once they had been approved by the directing committee and designed in conjunction with the operating body, could be carried out by qualified individuals in the Veterans Administration, medical colleges, or other appropriate institutions.[9]

On June 13, 1946, DeBakey and Beebe finished a draft of the report on the feasibility of a research program devoted to medical follow-up. Along with DeBakey's original memo, this report became one of the two founding documents of the Medical Follow-up Agency. A program of clinical research that focused on the follow-up of veterans would, the report said, make "a priceless contribution to clinical medicine," "stimulate research in clinical and scientific medicine," and "improve the level of medical practice in both federal and other hospitals." The National Research Council was the ideal place from which to run such an effort. As a quasi-government agency, it provided "the logical mechanism by which the resources of scientific and clinical medicine [could] be marshaled for the coordination and direction of so broad a program." Indeed, the program had to be broad enough to encompass clinical studies testing new therapies as well as statistical studies of mortality and morbidity. The report indicated "no insuperable barrier" to prevent the creation of rosters of people for studies, the use of wartime clinical records, or the location of people who would participate in follow-up activities. Bey ond these parameters, the report argued that the program could not be "visualized in definitive detail in advance of actual trial."[10]

FINDING THE FUNDING

One area of concern was funding for the new endeavor. The draft report recommended that no single agency provide all the funds, even though DeBakey and Beebe knew that the Veterans Administration was prepared to make a large contribution to the program. Even before the draft's completion, Paul R. Hawley, chief medical director of the Veterans Administration, announced his agency's intention to contract with the NRC for two types of services. At one level, the Veterans Administration desired help from the National Research Council with the direction of its extramural research, expecting the NRC to convene a supervisory committee for the research program and to issue contracts to the institutions carrying out the resulting research. The Veterans Administration also sought a follow-up program for which the NRC would provide "a statistical service to investigate military records and help in the development of research problems."

Pleased with this interest, DeBakey, Beebe, and the committee still saw the need for "broad financial participation" on the part of "all the interested federal medical agencies." They hoped that, at the least, the new entity would be headed by a "first-class medical executive" and would attract "medical analysts of the highest caliber." They wanted the new agency to be assured of five years of funding. Writing at a time when federal support for medical research through the National Institutes of Health had not yet become routine, they believed that this required access to nonfederal funds either as grants or "as guarantees against the failure of federal funds."[11]

The bottom-line recommendation was that the surgeons general and the VA's chief medical director should take steps that would enable the NRC's Division of Medical Sciences to establish "a continuing committee on clinical research and follow-up, with provision for administrative officers, professional and secretarial assistance . . . as well as funds for the support of a broadly conceived research program."[12] Beebe and DeBakey estimated that it would cost at least $200,000 to start the effort. As studies began, the annual amount needed would rise to $500,000. The report concluded with examples of the studies the new entity might undertake. These ranged from studies of infectious hepatitis to examinations of the personalities of military heroes.[13]

DeBakey and Beebe's draft report gained quick approval from the Committee on Veterans Medical Problems. Dr. Roy McClure of the Henry Ford Hospital in Detroit expressed positive "delight" with the proposed program, which he called "very sound." Advising the group not to change a word of the report, Dr. Paul Magnuson of the Veterans Administration said that "experience would indicate the necessary changes in due time." The priority was to get the program up and running. Toward this end, the committee endorsed the report with only minor modifications.[14]

2

The Early Committee Years

With the report in hand, the National Academy of Sciences (NAS) and the Veterans Administration (VA) entered into serious contract negotiations. By the end of summer 1946, the Academy had received promises of $850,000 from the VA for fiscal year 1946–1947. The money would establish a permanent Committee on Veterans Medical Problems (CVMP), maintain a central office in the National Research Council (NRC) devoted to medical follow-up activities, and subsidize research at veterans hospitals.[15]

The Academy set the enterprise in motion. In August, NRC and NAS officials agreed on a list of members for the permanent Committee on Veterans Medical Problems. The committee mostly consisted of faculty and researchers from prominent medical schools who had played key roles in the wartime medical effort and had been involved in the project's formulation. Although Dr. Edward Churchill was a committee member, he was no longer the chair. This responsibility fell to Dr. O.H. Perry Pepper of the University of Pennsylvania Medical School. Lewis Weed of the NRC told him that his duties would be light, involving only occasional meetings. Nonetheless, he and the committee faced a tremendous opportunity to "aid . . . the Veterans Administration in the betterment of the care of patients and in the conduct of follow-up studies on clinical cases which are the direct result of the World Wars."[16] On September 20, 1946, Dr. Pepper convened the permanent committee's first meeting.

By this time, the National Research Council had hired two staff members to direct the committee's work. Gilbert Beebe and John Ransmeir, M.D., became, in effect, the first Medical Follow-up Agency staff. Beebe handled matters related to statistics; Ransmeir supplied medical advice. Both were present at the first meeting.

8

From the beginning, a duality of purpose attended the committee's work. On the one hand, the committee was to advise the Veterans Administration on its medical programs. This advice involved matters related to clinical medical practice, such as whether radioactive isotopes should be used in VA hospitals. The VA also expected advice related to its research program. According to Paul Hawley, the VA was not equipped to undertake major clinical or biological studies. Instead of doing the work itself, it sought to fund extramural work that would be done in places with better facilities and superior personnel. Nor did VA officials feel competent to evaluate research proposals. The expectation was that the committee, along with other advisory committees of the NRC, such as those pertaining to medicine and neuropsychiatry, would handle this task.

The committee was also to serve as a focal point for follow-up studies that were not directly related to the VA's medical care. Hawley justified this by noting that the VA's greatest research contribution "would be the follow-up of disease conditions throughout a life-time or even throughout several generations." Dr. Francis Braceland also stressed that the committee should not allow its broad mission to cause it to lose sight of follow-up studies "as its major method of attack." The committee passed a motion that "in allocating support for research problems, emphasis be given to projects of major importance for long-term study."

FOLLOW-UP STUDIES

One study received consideration and approval at the committee's first meeting. The idea involved the study of soldiers from different geographic regions who had developed rheumatic fever during military service. A greater incidence of rheumatic fever among those in military service would suggest the importance of environment, rather than heredity. Control groups were formed by using adjacent serial numbers to choose from men with non-rheumatic fever hospital diagnoses in the same year or men who took out National Service Life Insurance, depending on the needs of the particular study. Affected soldiers were also to be compared with family members who had remained at home.

This study indicated just how useful the data gathered by the military could be in understanding the course of disease.[17] It also showed that follow-up could take many different forms. Michael DeBakey had tended to emphasize clinical follow-up: the reexamination of a patient to observe the course of a disease or the long-run efficacy of a particular treatment. Beebe, among others, had an interest in what he called "mass statistical studies," done entirely from records and not requiring a doctor to observe a patient. The most obvious sort of mass statistical study involved determining the death rates over time from individual diseases, injuries, or psychiatric conditions that had arisen during the war. Death records were widely available because an estimated 98 percent of all World War II veterans had taken out the National Service Life Insurance policies offered them during their service.[18]

Whether clinical or statistical, follow-up studies required the creation of rosters of people with particular diseases and demographic characteristics. Facilitating the creation of these rosters became a priority for Beebe and Ransmeir. If the rheumatic fever study was to be done, for example, it would require the creation of rosters that combined both medical and nonmedical characteristics of individuals. People in the rheumatic fever sample would have to be matched with controls with identical dates and places of induction, and identical training environments. The contemplated study would involve the medical records of up to 9,000 people. These records would have to be culled from the 18 million Army records housed in a federal records center in St. Louis, Missouri, which covered 1.5 million feet of floor space and employed 5,000 people. The Army eventually stationed teams of people working on follow-up studies approved by the NRC in the St. Louis center. Similar logistics had to be worked out with the Navy and the Veterans Administration. Eager to show that they could master their daunting task, Beebe and Ransmeir wanted to launch a pilot study that would locate and resolve the problems in the system of gathering records.[19] Traumatic epilepsy and arterial injuries were early candidates for such a study.

All in all, the work of the Committee on Veterans Medical Problems (CVMP) got under way in what the NRC described as a "deliberate and sensible fashion."[20] The committee began to receive and pass judgment on research proposals from other NRC advisory committees. Not all of the projects approved were follow-up studies. Some, including a study of group therapy in VA hospitals and clinics, merely happened to be conducted in VA facilities. Often, the follow-up studies that the committee approved came from investigators who had been involved in the committee's creation, as was the case with Barnes Woodhall's work on peripheral nerve injuries or DeBakey's follow-up of arterial injuries in veterans. After the first few years, the proposals came less often from other NRC committees and more often from outside sources such as university medical researchers.[21]

A project's approval meant little if funds were not available to support it. Almost immediately, the committee encountered problems caused by the uncertainties of federal funding. Although money was available to pay the salaries of Dr. Ransmeir and Dr. Beebe, who carried the respective titles of medical executive and medical statistician, funding for the studies proved more elusive to obtain. At the start of the 1948 fiscal year, the committee learned that extramural research money for the year had already been exhausted and the VA could not guarantee that funds would be available in fiscal year 1949.[22] In fact, the NRC had been given only two days to make a request for fiscal year 1948. The VA appealed to the Bureau of the Budget, but the bureau denied the request because of a lack of convincing documentation. Hence, the 1948 federal budget made no specific mention of the CVMP program and contained no provisions for contracts with universities or the NRC. The little money spent on CVMP projects came from a budget item designated for research by VA personnel in VA hospitals.[23]

The NRC blamed this situation on "current legislative uncertainties" concerning VA appropriations. Even with these difficulties, 20 projects approved by the CVMP were receiving VA funds in November 1947.[24] In the absence of funds for more projects, Beebe and Ransmeir worked on perfecting administrative routines, such as grant application procedures and the mechanics of preparing rosters from Army and Navy files. Beebe, in particular, collaborated with project directors on improving the statistical design of the projects.[25]

Throughout this early period, confusion persisted about the committee's mission. How much time and effort were to go to medical follow-up, and how much to other activities? Dr. Paul Magnuson of the VA noted that his agency already had a Board of Professional Consultants; presumably, the CVMP should serve a different function. Placing heavy emphasis on medical follow-up, he thought that the committee should concern itself primarily with the "salvage of medical information from our experience in the war and overall guidance and advice in the medical research program." Committee member Francis Braceland admitted that this aspect of the committee's work had developed slowly and should be "more actively pursued." DeBakey agreed but noted that funding was problematic. Because VA rules allowed contracts to be let for only a year at a time, an investigator had no assurance of continuing support. This was an important consideration in studies involving lengthy efforts to locate records, find the participants, perform clinical procedures, collect data, and assess the results. Dr. E.H. Cushing of the VA chastised the committee for routinely approving the suggestions of other committees and not coming up with ideas of its own. Cushing and others felt that the committee had not done enough to push the idea of medical follow-up.[26]

A curious duality in the committee's work emerged. In March 1948, the committee announced a significant "reorientation" in its "program and outlook"—from follow-up studies to what it described as "the entire medical research program of the Veterans Administration, of which the follow-up studies constitute merely one significant part." At the same time, however, the entity now known as the Medical Follow-up Agency began to take shape. At the end of 1947, for the first time, an entity distinct from the Committee on Veterans Medical Problems appeared on an NRC organizational chart. The committee had made a real start toward assembling the staff and facilities needed for the follow-up projects.

A change in personnel had occurred already. On March 20, 1948, Dr. Ransmeir resigned, and was replaced by Dr. Theodore Moise, a Johns Hopkins medical school graduate and surgeon with a background in bacteriology and pathology. Bernard M. Cohen, a Ph.D. statistician, also joined the organization, initially on a six-month loan from the Department of Commerce.[27] At the end of the year he was joined by Seymour Jablon, another applied mathematician. Both men, especially Jablon, would play major roles in the agency's history.

STARTING THE FOLLOW-UP AGENCY

On April 30, 1948, Gilbert Beebe reported for the first time to the Committee on Veterans Medical Problems on the operations of the Follow-up Agency. Although Beebe was sometimes described as director of the committee's statistical division, he had also become the agency's informal director. Its work included the statistical evaluation of all projects submitted by the committee, doing detailed statistical planning on clinical follow-up and mass statistical studies, assisting investigators in devising and testing record forms and schedules, drawing samples for studies, and providing investigators with data from service medical and personnel records. In little more than a year, the staff had done statistical planning for 16 follow-up studies. By this time the agency had three people working in the Records Center at St. Louis, and the VA had set aside space for the committee's operations in Washington, D.C. All in all, the agency payroll covered 24 full-time and 4 part-time employees, including 7 people engaged in statistical analysis and 16 people who worked with the federal records. Beebe said that there was a need for more trained statisticians who could help investigators with the statistical design of their projects. He worried about the possibility of introducing bias into the experiments because of inadequate or inappropriate sampling techniques. Hearing the report, the committee voted its "strong support of the activities and functions of the follow-up agency."[28]

By the fall of 1948, the committee had received the first tentative results from its projects. One such project, which concerned the long-term effects of hepatitis, illustrated the difficulty of undertaking such studies. The study examined the incidence of infectious and postvaccinal hepatitis in the armed forces during World War II. More than 200,000 such cases were estimated to have occurred during this time period. Investigators sought to determine long-term residuals of viral hepatitis infection (e.g., cirrhosis and other forms of liver disease). In the course of this research, doctors had a difficult time getting study participants to come in for examination. Such impediments reduced the statistical validity of the study's findings.[29]

The question of getting people to appear for examinations became a point of contention between the committee and the Veterans Administration. In April 1949, the committee identified this as its greatest problem. Most of the research in the 17 active follow-up projects took place in university clinics and hospitals. Nothing compelled a person to appear for an examination. Gilbert Beebe complained that the VA's prestige and resources were not being used to encourage veterans to submit to these examinations. Without help from the VA, Beebe believed that no more than 60 to 80 percent of the men chosen for study would be examined. The committee pushed the Veterans Administration to help by linking the Follow-up Agency's work with the physical examinations that the VA performed for other purposes (e.g., to rate a veteran's disability). The VA, for its part, felt that such action would be a misuse of a sensitive aspect of social policy.

Veterans needed to be reassured that their disability pensions were based on objective medical evidence; the necessary medical examinations were not to become tools of social experimentation. As a result, although the committee lauded the Army and the Navy for their extensive help in locating records, it found the VA somewhat recalcitrant in supporting follow-up work. "Over the past two years repeated efforts to obtain more cooperation from the VA have not been successful," Dr. Perry Pepper lamented.[30]

The VA had its own grievances with the committee. At a time of rapid expansion of the National Institutes of Health (NIH), the leaders of the VA felt that they were losing influence in the medical research establishment. They believed that the NRC, which received support from the VA, should be a stronger advocate for its patron. The VA also believed that the committee made decisions too slowly and, in the process, encouraged researchers to seek funds from the NIH and other parts of the Public Health Service. Cushing, the VA's assistant medical director for research and education, asserted that if the NRC did not provide better service, the VA would set up its own advisory committees.[31]

Beebe, Cohen, and others in the agency turned their attention toward studies that substituted paper records for the direct medical observation of individuals. As a test of this method, they attempted to see how many cases in a given roster of veterans could be located through Veterans Administration records, or other means, and discovered that they were able to trace a high percentage of people in the various groups. Of a group of 403 World War II veterans with Hodgkin's disease, for example, they were able to trace 384, or 88.5 percent. They concluded that "if the test of feasibility of these studies is a demonstration that every man on a roster can be accounted for until he dies, . . . the results so far indicate that it is possible to come very close to such an accounting."[32] With such information, many studies of mortality, morbidity, and disability became possible. One could, for example, compare survival rates for different diseases over time.[33] For this reason, the committee endorsed a program of mass statistical studies, hoping that certain diseases could be followed routinely for mortality, morbidity, and rates of hospitalization.[34]

By the end of the 1940s, the Committee on Veterans Medical Problems and the Follow-up Agency had acquired a new degree of sophistication. The committee rarely accepted an application for a study unless its staff had explored the study's administrative and statistical feasibility. Adding mathematical statistician Jablon to the staff removed some of the burden from Beebe in the performance of such work. Record follow-up studies, those that did not involve a clinical examination, were made easier by the appointment of Bernard Cohen on a permanent basis. Ms. Nona Murray Lucke, an experienced record executive, helped in gathering data from the various archives in which it was stored. Regina Loewenstein supervised statistical coding, tabulation, and analysis. These staffers made it possible for clinical work on various projects to take place in 30 different centers around the nation.[35]

THE FIRST ROUND OF STUDIES

By the spring of 1950, five of the seven projects approved in 1947 were nearing completion. These included studies of psychoneurosis, peripheral nerve injuries, vascular injuries (see photo), and infectious hepatitis. Of the 19 clinical follow-up studies being conducted during fiscal year 1950, observations had been completed in 8 of them. The initial round of studies had taken longer to complete and was more expensive than investigators had originally contemplated. Most of the investigators had budgeted for only the clinical phase of the project and would need additional funds for the data analysis to follow. Despite these financial issues, the work of the Committee on Veterans Medical Problems had already generated 59 published papers related to the various studies.[36]

As the first round of studies neared completion attention turned toward the next steps. Neither Gilbert Beebe nor any of his staff had envisioned such a large program. Each project turned out to be time-consuming, and 20 active projects put a severe strain on staff resources. Still, they needed to recruit new projects to

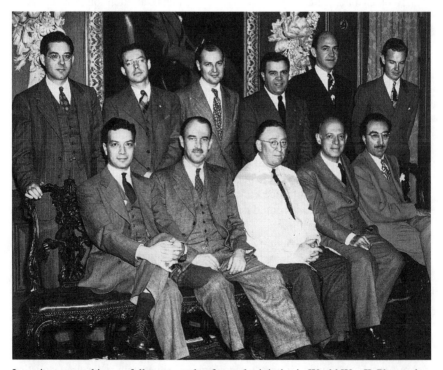

Investigators working on follow-up study of vascular injuries in World War II. Photo taken at Emory University in Atlanta, circa 1950. Dr. Gilbert Beebe, second from left, back row; Dr. Michael DeBakey, far right, front row. Photo courtesy of Dr. Gilbert Beebe.

replace the old ones. This process had to take place with full regard for both scientific rigor and the usual vagaries of the budget process. In fiscal year 1950, for example, the Bureau of the Budget reduced the VA's budget for research contracts from the requested $2.9 million to $1.8 million. Another problem that the committee faced concerned reporting the results of the first studies. Beebe hoped that there would be "careful analysis" of the statistical data, not simply a reporting of results. For projects that were spread among several medical centers, care would have to be taken to ensure that the publication of results was coordinated across centers. The committee hoped it would have the chance to examine each manuscript "for statistical review" before publication.[37]

Among the projects that the Committee on Veterans Medical Problems considered during this period was one devoted to capturing the long-term outcomes of people who had sustained trench foot, immersion foot, or frostbite in World War II. To facilitate this project, Beebe obtained rosters from the Veterans Administration and the Army. Five centers would examine about 100 patients from the 115 patients' files that they would be given. The sampling plan allowed each center to see a disproportionate number of severe cases. Although the study would not yield exact information on the effect of individual forms of treatment, "residuals of cold injury" would be obtained and related to the severity of the original injury. To minimize variance in the clinical examinations, doctors in New Orleans examined ten cases in advance of the study and obtained satisfactory agreement on their observations. DeBakey, still an active member of the CVMP, observed that although expensive, the study would provide "much needed information on the natural history of this condition." The committee recommended that $67,187 be given to the principal investigators for this study.[38]

Dr. F.A. Simeone, an investigator in the cold injury study, had already participated in a study of veterans who had incurred arterial wounds. In this latter study, he continued work that he had done during the war. For example, he had treated one patient by means of "non-suture anastomosis," reencountered the patient during the follow-up study, and found the patient to be symptom-free. The project also enabled him to follow up other patients who had received similar treatment to determine how many of them complained of intermittent claudication (irregular gait) or pain in walking. His preliminary observation was that sympathectomy, defined as the transection, resection, or other interruption of some portion of the sympathetic nervous pathways, decreased the incidence of claudication. Although the technical terms made the discussion difficult for non-doctors to follow, the process demonstrated that the agency's initial work followed directly from clinical interests that doctors had developed during the war.[39]

IMPACT OF THE KOREAN WAR

Beginning in 1950, the Korean War changed the tone of the follow-up program. What had been a leisurely excursion into the medical records from the

Second World War now acquired a new sense of urgency as administrators tried to determine what lessons from the previous war they could apply to the present one.

The outbreak of war added new funding pressures to the program. In particular, Dr. E.H. Cushing of the Veterans Administration wanted to know whether the follow-up program was cost-effective. Accordingly, the Committee on Veterans Medical Problems, now headed by Dr. Wilbert C. Davison, a professor of pediatrics and dean of the medical school at Duke, created an ad hoc committee to investigate the follow-up program's cost and value. The committee included himself, Michael DeBakey (at the time chairman of the department of surgery at Baylor), Dr. Allen O. Whipple of New York's Memorial Hospital, and Herbert Marks of the Metropolitan Life Insurance Company.[40]

On January 22, 1951, the ad hoc committee reported to Cushing and Dr. Milton C. Winternitz, chairman of the NRC's Division of Medical Sciences. "All of us have expected concrete, tangible, and useful results from the VA follow-up projects but none of us realized, until the meeting today, how excellent the progress has been and how important the reports are even in their preliminary stage," Davison wrote. He predicted that the VA, the military, and the taxpayers would "all profit enormously" if the program was continued.[41]

Many findings presented at the meeting illustrated the wide reach of the program; two of the most important concerned hepatitis and schizophrenia. In the hepatitis study, a follow-up of approximately 1,000 survivors of infectious hepatitis revealed no residual or severe liver damage. In the schizophrenia study, the average length of service prior to breakdown was two and a half years. Investigators concluded that the majority of cases could have been detected by adequate study at time of induction.[42]

In the short run, the findings that mattered most were those that appeared to have relevance to the Korean War situation. Herbert Marks noted that the tuberculosis studies would help the armed forces weed out men who were likely to come down with this disease, reducing the loss of manpower in the field and the costs of pensions and medical care. The studies of peripheral nerve and arterial injuries led to more effective management of these types of casualties in Korea. As DeBakey noted, the finding that there were no long-term consequences of infectious hepatitis once a patient recovered from the disease would affect the determination of disability pensions for both wars. DeBakey admitted that the work was "costly and time-consuming" but noted that "the preliminary reports of some of the studies already provide knowledge that should permit great savings in the operational activities of the Veterans Administration."[43]

The review of follow-up activities that took place at the beginning of the Korean War enabled the Committee on Veterans Medical Problems and the Follow-up Agency to gain a comprehensive view of the work being undertaken. Each investigator submitted a report that summarized a study's findings and outlined preliminary conclusions. From a study of posttraumatic epilepsy came the finding that 20.9 percent of a sample of men who had suffered head wounds had epileptic seizures. Most of the epilepsy developed within the first two years of the injury. A large study of 2,700 men with peripheral nerve injuries (see summary of study in Box 1), conducted at five university hospitals, reinforced the necessity for specialized neurologic treatment of such injuries, including early diagnosis, prompt evacuation, and the use of special neurophysiological techniques as an adjunct to surgery. A follow-up study of schistosomiasis acquired during military service revealed that a majority of patients still complained of such symptoms as diarrhea, abdominal cramps, right-upper-quadrant pain, and fatigue. A study of rheumatic fever, in contrast, demonstrated no progression of the disease for at least five to seven years after the attack that occurred during service.[44]

In the spring of 1951, the CVMP reported that investigations of psychoneurosis, tuberculosis, hepatitis, sarcoidosis, and testicular tumors were ending. Follow-up studies of peripheral nerve injuries, vascular injuries, schistosomiasis, and schizophrenia were close to completion. In order to do the statistical analysis for these studies, the follow-up staff decreased the amount of time it spent locating records, thus restricting its ability to start new studies. The intent was to produce information that would be useful to the military in the Korean effort (e.g., management of particular types of wounds, induction policy) as quickly as

---

Box 1
Study of Peripheral Nerve Injury

In 1957, the Medical Follow-up Agency (MFUA) and its collaborators published a study of peripheral nerve regeneration based on the follow-up of 3,656 World War II injuries. Clinical follow-up data for this study, one of the first proposed to the Committee on Veterans Medical Problems, were gathered at five clinical centers (in Chicago, Boston, New York, Philadelphia, and San Francisco), all of which followed a standardized data-gathering protocol. Three-quarters of the men in the study eventually reported for examination and participated in the study.

The study determined the optimal time for nerve suture and established the value of physical therapy during the time of nerve regeneration. For nerve injury with total loss of function, the study suggested that a radical approach should be used, whereas for cases in which the continuity of a nerve has not been interrupted, treatment should be conservative, with end-to-end suture substituted for neurolysis. In addition, functional recovery was shown to be reasonably predictable on the basis of the distance from the lesion to its area of principal innervation.

Selected Reference

Woodhall, B., Beebe, G.W. Peripheral Nerve Regeneration, a Follow-up Study of 3,656 World War II Injuries. VA Medical Monograph. Washington, D.C.: U.S. Government Printing Office, 1957.

possible. Only the cold injury study was added to the clinical follow-up program during fiscal year 1951, and the agency sacrificed the expansion of "record follow-up studies" (those that did not involve clinical observations) in order to complete the clinical studies. The military emergency in Korea also made it more difficult for the agency to obtain the equipment necessary for its work, such as the IBM machines "best suited to the kind of work performed."[45]

During this period, Gilbert Beebe began giving speeches in which he described the Follow-up Agency's mission to military and medical audiences. In these talks, he put forth questions that the agency sought to answer, such as: Do men with severe frostbite and trench foot recover completely? or What is the chance of survival for men with Hodgkin's disease? He emphasized the value of military records for scientific investigation. "If you want a thousand cases of schistosomiasis, there is a specific place to go and you can physically put your hands on a thousand punchcards which represent a thousand admissions for this disease," he said. He claimed that "everyone has felt much better . . . knowing that a single group has been entrusted with the responsibility of organizing access to this material and of evaluating the specific research proposals made in connection with it." As for the investigators who worked with this material, Beebe cited a group of committed doctors who had become interested in a particular problem during the war and who were willing "to put up with a considerable amount of necessary administrative and organizational work" in order to use the records. However, even the most committed clinical investigators required the help of agency staff in acquiring rosters, locating individuals, and examining sample records, and even then, considerable problems remained in getting people to report for examinations. Still, concluded Beebe, the rewards of such an enterprise were immense.[46]

Despite Beebe's optimism, the future of the follow-up program was far from ensured. Between 1952 and 1955, the agency faced a painful transition from total dependence on the Veterans Administration to more diverse sources of financial support. This period coincided with expansion of the VA's own intramural activities, which decreased its reliance on external contracts, and with the arrival of the first Republican administration in Washington since 1932.

In a statement prepared in April 1952, Gilbert Beebe wrote that until final reports were prepared for some of the larger and more expensive studies, it would be difficult to "know whether the program should be brought to an end as a post-war episode of temporary interest and value." At the end of fiscal year 1952, total costs for the effort were expected to reach $2.2 million, with about 38 percent going to the Follow-up Agency itself. The most expensive of the 25 projects cost $600,000. Beebe admitted that the conduct of cooperative, multicenter projects had proved to be a challenge. Even within single centers, the staff noted that well-qualified examiners differed greatly in their reports "as to specific signs, symptoms, and laboratory values." These diagnostic differences, coupled with the agency's inability to compel individuals to submit to examination, revealed tensions between the exacting world of the statistician and the pragmatic concerns of the clinician.[47]

Responding to the financial problems and the mounting concerns of the Veterans Administration, the Committee on Veterans Medical Problems decided that each follow-up project would be studied by experts on the particular subject, with the objective of assessing the report's "value."[48] Five years of effort had, according to Dr. Winternitz, brought "relatively little harvest to date." The NRC wanted to evaluate the follow-up program through the final reports of the various studies, but "unfortunately," noted Winternitz, none of the major studies had been completed. Beebe said that the slow pace of the work reflected the many stages of a project. Even after the clinical examinations had been performed, agency staff still needed to perform the tabulations, conduct the statistical analysis, work with the investigator on a final manuscript, and make a final check of the statistics and tables used in the manuscript. Beebe hoped that the bulk of the statistical work on approved projects would be completed by the end of June 1953.[49] In the meantime, the majority of the committee's work shifted from the follow-up studies to advising the Veterans Administration on its intramural research program.[50]

REVIEWING THE AGENCY'S PROGRESS

By early 1953, the follow-up studies program was officially under "review and reassessment" by the NRC. The reasons were both internal and external. The Agency staff was overloaded with statistical work. Some of the investigators were late with their final reports. With the arrival of President Dwight D. Eisenhower and a Republican Congress, the external environment was also changing. The Veterans Administration faced a stringent review of its budget requests. President Eisenhower proposed the creation of a cabinet-level Department of Health, Education, and Welfare (HEW) that would include the Public Health Service and possibly other medical programs of the federal government, including those of the VA as well. Beebe and others feared the impact that the new HEW would have on the agency's funding relationships with the federal government.[51]

Although the work of the Follow-up Agency appeared to be stalled, the staff enjoyed a period of considerable creativity and productivity. Bernard Cohen continued his work on the studies in which he made use of existing medical records to illuminate larger epidemiological and policy concerns. His pilot study, begun in 1948 and designated R-1 or record study one, led to a detailed draft final report in 1951 (draft because it had to be put aside in the crush of other work) and to a summary of the methodology, which was published in the *American Journal of Public Health*, the first of a long series of staff publications that became the agency's hallmark. The success of this project encouraged the agency to undertake other record studies, each involving Cohen and one of his colleagues, on subjects such as Hodgkin's disease, tuberculosis, prisoners or war, and Buerger's disease (thromboangiitis obliterans).

The prisoner of war study (see Box 2), designated R-4, which was to focus a great deal of attention on the agency, involved examining an environmental situation rather than a disease entity, for which the record approach was better suited than the clinical approach. The study itself focused on the mortality expe-

---

BOX 2
Mortality Studies of Former Prisoners of War

Almost as old as the Medical Follow-up Agency (MFUA) is the series of follow-up studies, now seven in number, of former prisoners of war (POW) from World War II and the Korean War. Some of the studies have focused on mortality and others on morbidity (see Box 8). Work began with a study, published in 1955, which presented findings on mortality, morbidity, and disability after liberation, as well the recollections of prison experience. The study showed, for example, that former POWs of the Japanese suffered markedly higher mortality, due primarily to tuberculosis and accidents, following their repatriation than did a group of comparison veterans; this was not the case for prisoners of the Germans.

In the second study of the series, the original sample was augmented through the addition of POWs from the Korean War and combat comparison individuals, as well as a group of malnourished World War II POWs. This brought the mortality sample to more than 19,000 men and the morbidity sample, which was smaller because morbidity follow-up was more expensive, to more than 5,000. By the time of the study, which was published in 1970, the excess mortality among World War II Pacific prisoners, relative to the U.S. general population, had practically disappeared, whereas the mortality rate of POWs of the Korean War remained significantly higher than that of the U.S. population for more than a decade.

The results of the next mortality study, the fourth overall, were published in 1975. It was clear by this time that the early increased risk of dying among former POWs had waned, although excess deaths due to cirrhosis of the liver appeared as a late effect.

As the MFUA entered its sixth decade, a seventh study of former POWs was begun. This mortality study will provide 50 years of follow-up data, capping the literally decades-long MFUA efforts.

Selected References

Cohen, B.M., Cooper, M.Z. A Follow-up Study of World War II Prisoners of War. VA Medical Monograph. Washington, D.C.: U.S. Government Printing Office, 1955.

Keehn, R.J. Follow-up studies of World War II and Korean Conflict prisoners. III. Mortality to 1 January 1976. *American Journal of Epidemiology* 111:194–211, 1980.

Nefzger, M.D. Follow-up studies of World War II and Korean War prisoners. I. Study plan and mortality findings. *American Journal of Epidemiology* 91:123–138, 1970.

rience of the prisoners. Preliminary computations indicated that those who had been prisoners of war in Japan experienced an excess of mortality compared to the U.S. white male population in the period between 1945 and 1951; prisoners in Europe had a significantly lower mortality rate than U.S. white males for this period. Excited by this finding, the staff believed that record follow-up projects deserved a more important place in the committee program than they had received. As Bernard Cohen put it, "the medical records of the armed forces and the Veterans Administration provide unparalleled materials and opportunities for follow-up studies."[52]

Donald Mainland, a professor of medical statistics at New York University, produced a more sober evaluation of the Follow-up Agency in a report for the NRC that appeared in March 1953. He lauded the work of Gilbert Beebe and his staff. Still, he found much to criticize. In the excitement at the beginning of the program, studies had begun without sufficient planning. Few people understood that clinical competence did not imply statistical competence. The agency did not do enough small pilot studies. Instead, it undertook too many large projects, too quickly. The clinical investigators failed to appreciate the importance of statistical expertise. All in all, the relative value of the program would have been greater "if those responsible (investigators and committee members) had been better acquainted with the principles and limitations of statistical surveys." Mainland argued that if the program continued, it should do so on a diminished scale. In the meantime, the NRC might consider establishing a statistical advisory unit to serve a wide variety of purposes.[53]

With Mainland's report in hand, the Committee on Veterans Medical Problems discussed the future of the follow-up program in April 1953. The committee decided that applications for new follow-up studies should have an adequate experimental plan, an estimate of the "feasibility of the proposal from a statistical viewpoint," and investigators "with enthusiasm, competence, and dependability in regard to completion of the study." In other words, they proposed to interpret existing standards in a rigorous manner. The committee looked with particular skepticism on projects that involved multiple research locations.[54]

3

Changing Times

The future of the Follow-up Agency remained unresolved. During a May 1953 meeting of the Executive Committee of the National Research Council's (NRC's) Division of Medical Sciences, Dr. Milton Winternitz reiterated that the follow-up program was under "critical review."[55] At the division's annual meeting, Dr. Wilbert Davison noted that a careful evaluation of the follow-up studies had been under way for a year and that the number of applications received by his committee had decreased. He added that the Veterans Administration (VA) continued to place greater emphasis on intramural research.[56] In a private June meeting with Dr. R. Keith Cannan, soon to become the new chairman of the Division of Medical Sciences, Gilbert Beebe encountered a "neutral, show me" attitude. Cannan asked Beebe to make a case for the agency's continuation at the October meeting of the Executive Committee.[57]

At this meeting, members of the Executive Committee learned that the interest in follow-up studies was diminishing. Unless the VA showed greater interest or other funding agencies came forward, it would be necessary to consider "a progressive scaling-down and ultimate termination of the operation." Furthermore, the program had a "chequered history" because it attempted too many projects at once.[58] Meanwhile, the Veterans Administration's 1954 research budget had been cut from a requested $6.5 million to $5.5 million and the number of the VA's own research laboratories had tripled in three years. In such a situation, any external research program that depended on VA funds would face difficulties. The follow-up program had received nearly $2.5 million from the VA over seven years, and had spent the bulk of it on clinical research done in 40 universities. The peripheral nerve injury study alone had absorbed about a quarter of the funds. Listening to Beebe and Michael DeBakey defend the basic concept of follow-up studies, the Executive Committee agreed that "the medical experience of the Armed Forces and of the veteran population provide[d] a unique opportunity for . . . studies of importance to clinical medicine and to the Armed Forces and the Veterans Administration." It decided that "steps should be taken to re-establish, as a broad inter-agency program, a significant program of medical follow-up studies."[59]

The Follow-up Agency had won a reprieve and a chance for survival if it could raise funds from sources other than the VA. If, as Keith Cannan and other NRC officials fully expected, a follow-up program of "carefully selected studies" could be justified, then the NRC would make an "intensive effort" to underwrite the program.[60] Encouraged, the Committee on Veterans Medical Problems recommended that the VA continue its financial support of the Follow-up Agency "to the fullest extent of its ability even though this mean[t] that other parts of the extramural contractual program [might] have to be curtailed."

In the meantime, the committee urged the NRC to "continue efforts to acquire multiple agency support."[61] With the Korean War ending and interest in civilian medical research booming, it now appeared logical to deemphasize studies of military concern and highlight "general medical interests in the natural history of disease."[62]

With this new mandate, the Follow-up Agency set out to win contracts from the many federal and private agencies that funded medical research. Although initial discussions about funding individual projects went well, money to maintain the central staff proved more difficult to obtain. The NRC estimated that a reserve of $50,000 to $70,000 in unrestricted funds would be necessary for this purpose.[63] The NRC looked to the Department of Defense, the National Institutes of Health (NIH), and the American Cancer Society as possible benefactors. Cannan summarized the situation in March 1954: "The efforts of the Follow-up Agency to enlist the cooperation of a number of agencies in a program of cogent investigations are meeting with encouraging success." The agency expected to gather a nucleus of direct support from the Army for the study of epidemic hemorrhagic fever, and from the National Institutes of Health for the follow-up of approximately 1,000 patients with Buerger's disease and 100,000 naval recruits with tuberculosis (see Box 3). The possibility of contractual support from the VA existed as well.[64]

By November 1954, the Follow-up Agency had assisted in the publication of reports from its initial round of studies and had initiated three new projects. Papers on such subjects as psychoneurosis, schizophrenia, viral hepatitis, fractures of the carpal scaphoid, wounds of the hand, testicular tumors, rheumatic fever, sarcoidosis, and the aftereffects of million-volt x-ray all reflected research that had been done under the auspices of the Committee on Veterans Medical Problems. As for new projects, the National Heart Institute supported Michael DeBakey and Bernard Cohen's study of Buerger's disease, which consisted of a

---

BOX 3
Studies of Tuberculosis

In 1955, a study was published by the Medical Follow-up Agency (MFUA) and its collaborators comparing induction and separation x-ray films for roughly 3,000 veterans who were discharged from military service because of tuberculosis (TB) and 3,000 control veterans who were not discharged for this reason. The researchers found that about half of the men discharged from military service because of TB had had the disease in x-ray-detectable form at induction. The films themselves did not always provide an evident reason why lesions on the induction x-ray appear to have been overlooked, but it was noted that failures of detection were greater at stations known to have inferior medical service. The rate of apparently new cases of tuberculosis developed in service was found to be nearly twice as high among nonwhite as among white men, and tall, thin men developed tuberculosis more frequently. In addition, former prisoners of war had an excessively high rate of tuberculosis.

In the fall of 1957, a study of tuberculosis morbidity in Navy recruits was published. The data came from a multiple skin-testing program carried out between 1949 and 1951 in San Diego, California. Data were available for nearly 70,000 young men. One of the two goals of the study was to provide nationwide data on the prevalence of sensitivity to tuberculin antigen; the other was to determine the number of new tuberculosis cases following testing. As part of the second goal, the incidence of TB among those who had a positive reaction to the skin test was to be compared to its incidence among nonreactors.

Investigators found an average annual incidence rate of TB of 40 per 100,000, with a rate of 29 per 100,000 in the nonreactors and 157 per 100,000 in the reactors (a positive reaction was defined as one in which the induration measured 10 mm or more across). Height or weight did not appear to be associated with tuberculin reactivity, although lighter men did have a significantly higher rate of TB than heavier men. The study further determined that the value of x-ray screening for tuberculosis among those with an unequivocably negative tuberculin reactivity test was questionable.

Selected References

Long, E.R., Jablon, S. Tuberculosis in the Army of the United States in World War II: An Epidemiological Study with an Evaluation of X-Ray Screening. VA Medical Monograph. Washington, D.C.: U.S. Government Printing Office, 1955.
Palmer, A.E., Jablon, S., Edwards, P.Q. Tuberculosis morbidity of young men in relation to tuberculin sensitivity and body build. *American Review of Tuberculosis* 76:517–539, 1957.

---

record follow-up of a large number of Army hospital admissions for this disease between 1942 and 1948. The U.S. Public Health Service funded Seymour Jablon's study of tuberculosis in naval recruits. The agency also participated in a clinical experiment, funded by the VA and conducted in ten VA hospitals, studying treatment of multiple sclerosis with the drug isoniazid. This was the first multicentered, randomized, double-blind treatment trial carried out in the study of multiple sclerosis.[65] In addition to these studies, four others, including one by Cohen on the incidence of cancer in veterans, remained active possibilities.

Each of these new studies demonstrated that agency staff was taking a more active role in writing proposals and conducting research. No longer did the agency wait for proposals to reach the Committee on Veterans Medical Problems (CVMP). As a consequence, members of the agency staff began to develop expertise in particular areas and to publish more papers. In 1954, for example, a paper that appeared in the *Journal of the American Medical Association* on the sequelae of rheumatic fever carried only the name of Ephraim Engleman, the principal investigator who had received a grant from the committee, and his collaborators. In contrast, a monograph on the follow-up of World War II prisoners of war went to press under the names of agency staffer Bernard Cohen and an investigator from the VA.[66]

The new emphasis on entrepreneurial activity made Gilbert Beebe uncomfortable. He realized that the competence of the group he had assembled lay in methodology. The staff functioned best when someone brought them a problem to solve. In the changed circumstances of the mid-1950s, the members of the CVMP were no longer supplying the staff with projects. This required staff members to go out and sell their services, as Beebe put it, "to those who might have appropriate problems to solve."

The agency also faced an age-old dilemma encountered by nonprofit agencies: no project funds could be obtained until planning had been done, but no support was available for planning activities. As the NIH's James Shannon pointed out, the agency needed a specific program with specific objectives, but Beebe resisted this notion. His group, he believed, was not equipped to identify scientific problems or assess their importance. In the end, the agency functioned best when it facilitated the work of others or engaged in collaborative enterprises with clinical researchers.[67]

The decline in extramural research support from the VA affected not only the Follow-up Agency but its parent committee as well. Dr. Theodore S. Moise, who had been the NRC's chief staff officer to the Committee on Veterans Medical Problems and the only medical doctor who worked with the committee, resigned to take a position with the Veterans Administration. With his departure, the committee faced a period of reorganization, since its primary purpose, to award research contracts, no longer occupied much of its time.[68] Since the Follow-up Agency received most of its funds from agencies other than the VA, it no longer made as much sense for the Committee on Veterans Medical Problems to supervise it. Beebe worked to assemble a more informal steering group, composed of representatives from the NRC, the VA, the National Cancer Institute, and the armed forces. This group, it was hoped, would provide a forum for problems faced by one or more of the agencies for which "the records resources of the cooperating agencies provide the best means of attack."[69] Under this arrangement, the CVMP would continue to advise the VA on projects that required access to VA records, but a prolonged slippage in its influence with the Veterans Administration began.[70]

By the end of 1955, the survival of the Follow-up Agency appeared to be ensured. The budget for fiscal year 1956 totaled $120,000 after overhead. Although the VA continued to be the largest single financial sponsor, the Public Health Service and the Army each contributed almost as much. The budget guaranteed the agency's continuation, but it barely covered the more than 21 individuals whom the agency hoped to retain, including 4 professional statisticians and 17 clerical and technical personnel.[71]

The core staff found itself pulled in many different directions. Staff members participated actively in designing current projects, including a study of the incidence of cancer in veterans, a follow-up on fractures of the femur that had been treated in the European and Mediterranean theaters of operation, and a study of the mortality rates of World War I veterans exposed to mustard gas or post-influenzal pneumonia. They also collaborated with doctors in universities and the government on final reports for completed projects. In this role, Bernard Cohen worked with Dr. H.F. Smetana of the Armed Forces Institute of Pathology on a report dealing with the course of Hodgkin's disease from onset to death, and Jablon applied the final statistical touches to a report concerning head injuries sustained in World War II (see Box 4). Gilbert Beebe completed a collaborative report on "variations in psychological tolerance to ground combat." Cohen, Jablon, and Beebe were also in the process of reviewing manuscripts on the subjects of prisoners of war and tuberculosis in the Army. Even as they undertook these activities, they also explored the possibility of starting new projects such as creating a roster of twins, which later emerged as a central activity for the agency, and studying the natural history of hypertension.[72]

As the core staff did more, the Committee on Veterans Medical Problems did less. It still met several times a year and discussed each of the major studies being considered by the Follow-up Agency. The CVMP officially recommended whether Veterans Administration records should be used for a particular study. With a study proposed by Bernard Cohen on coronary heart disease in young adult males, the committee faced a situation in which the project had already been reviewed favorably by the National Advisory Heart Council. This meant that the study would be funded by NIH. Still, the committee found it necessary to review the proposal with an eye toward "the propriety and desirability" of granting the investigators access to VA records.[73] The committee also contemplated procedures that had proved troublesome from the very beginning of the program. In June 1956, for example, it responded to a complaint from Dr. Barnes Woodhall about the difficulty in getting patients to come to the hospital to participate in follow-up studies. He argued that the Veterans Administration should use its authority to compel people to appear, but how to do so was unclear. The resulting discussion ended as had many similar discussions. The committee reached no conclusion and took no action.

BOX 4
Studies of Head Injury

A paper published in the *Journal of Neurosurgery* (see Walker and Jablon, 1959) documented the work of the Medical Follow-up Agency and its collaborators on the study of head wounds in World War II; this publication was later followed (Walker and Jablon, 1961) by a book-length monograph. The material on which these reports were based came from examinations of 739 World War II veterans with head wounds who appeared at one of four clinical centers in Baltimore, New York, Boston, or Long Beach. The most common wound was a penetrating wound of the brain (i.e., a compound, comminuted fracture).

Mental disturbances, such as impaired judgment and altered personality, were found to be related to the extent of injury, but not to its location, whereas aphasia (impaired production or comprehension of speech) was present when right-handed patients had been wounded in the left hemisphere of the brain. Headache, present in 82 percent of the men, was not correlated with the severity of injury.

Whereas 28 percent of the men examined suffered from epilepsy, only 23 percent were found to have had multiple attacks. Wounds of increased diameter and depth were found to be associated with higher rates of epilepsy, particularly with multiple focal attacks. Similarly, a longer duration of unconsciousness after receiving a wound was related to increased risk of epilepsy. However, neurological symptoms at the time of wounding were not associated with later epilepsy. Finally, men who had their first epileptic attack sooner after receiving a wound had a more favorable prognosis than those whose first attack occurred later.

Selected References

Walker, E.A., Jablon, S. A follow-up of head-injured men of World War II. *Journal of Neurosurgery* 16:600–610, 1959.

Walker, E.A., Jablon, S. A Follow-up Study of Head Wounds in World War II. VA Medical Monograph. Washington, D.C.: U.S. Government Printing Office, 1961.

NEW PROJECTS IN THE LATE 1950s

The June 1956 meeting featured the first extended discussion of the study of twins. The project came to the agency's attention in 1955 through Dr. William B. Wartman of Northwestern University. As early as 1953, Beebe had identified the veteran population as a valuable resource for twin studies. Together, Bernard Cohen and Seymour Jablon explored the feasibility of creating a roster of twins. They discovered that a roster of as many as 10,000 pairs of twins could be developed from military records. It would, however, involve a great deal of effort and would not be cost-effective unless the roster could be used over a long period of time for many studies. Jablon estimated that each pair of veteran twins would cost between five and ten dollars to identify. The laborious process would involve checking with vital statistics authorities in each state to obtain a list of twins born during the period that made them likely to have served in the armed forces during World War II. The list would then have to be checked against military records to see if a particular set of twins did, in fact, enlist. This method was cheaper than beginning with the military records and then checking to see if two servicemembers with the same last name were actually twins. To perform experiments that tried to discriminate between the effects of environment and heredity, it would also be necessary to separate the sample into monozygotic and dizygotic pairs (fraternal and identical twins). Jablon believed that, by using physical characteristics such as eye color, hair color, height, weight, and complexion, as well as fingerprints (obtained from the Federal Bureau of Investigation [FBI]), he could make accurate classifications in 80 percent of the cases.[74] The committee expressed enthusiasm for the project, provided that a source of funds could be found.

The Follow-up Agency sought external advice from Dr. James Neel of the University of Michigan's Institute of Human Biology, who advised Bernard Cohen that, in an ideal situation, one would like to be able to observe the twins from birth to the grave. A sample of twins from Veterans Administration records would eliminate the first and much of the second decade of life and would not contain many people with congenital defects who, presumably, would have been screened out in the induction process. Hence, the sample would not be of much use in studying congenital malformations or the malignant diseases of childhood such as leukemia. Yet Neel believed the sample "would certainly be far better than anything that the world has ever had before."[75]

Beginning in 1957, Neel chaired an ad hoc committee on studies of veteran twins that gave the NRC and the Follow-up Agency still more advice on the project. It became a permanent institution in the Follow-up Agency and continued the ongoing separation of the agency and the Committee on Veterans Medical Problems by removing much of the twin study oversight from the committee. At the first meeting, after a lengthy discussion of such technical matters as determining zygosity (i.e., whether the twins were identical or fraternal), the ad hoc committee reached the same positive conclusion as the CVMP. It recommended that "steps be taken to establish a roster of twin veterans as soon as possible." As soon as the roster was established, the committee suggested that the agency undertake a pilot study to compare the relative effectiveness of various diagnostic methods for establishing zygosity.[76]

Although the study of twins appeared to set the Follow-up Agency off in a new direction, Gilbert Beebe hesitated to loosen the ties with the Committee on Veterans Medical Problems. His staff, he realized, focused on methodology, not specific medical subjects. Stimulus for selecting specific subjects had to come from external investigators, and the agency needed the committee's help in making connections with such researchers. The agency, Beebe noted, had ready access to records, not to investigators.

In 1957, another important development occurred when Keith Cannan asked the agency to participate in the program of the Atomic Bomb Casualty Commission (ABCC; Box 5). Seymour Jablon became the first staff member to go to

BOX 5
Studies of Atomic Bomb Survivors

The world was introduced to the atomic age in 1945 when bombs devastated Hiroshima and, a few days later, Nagasaki, Japan. Japanese scientists soon arrived and began to investigate and assess the physical damage, deaths, and injuries among inhabitants and the effects on survivors. The occupation forces dispatched their own teams, which combined with the Japanese on the scene to form a joint commission to investigate the effects of the bombings. Impressed with the obvious magnitude of this task and the time that would be required to complete it, President Truman, in a November 1946 executive order, asked the National Academy of Sciences to undertake a program, funded by the Atomic Energy Commission (now the Department of Energy), to study the long-range biological and medical effects of the atomic bomb on man. Thus was born the Atomic Bomb Casualty Commission (ABCC).

Guided by existing information from studies of mice about the health and genetic effects of radiation, James V. Neel inaugurated large-scale genetic studies of the offspring of survivors. Other investigators sent by the Academy did not, however, recognize that a strong, long-term, epidemiologic effort would be needed; hence, no comprehensive plan was implemented. The major early emphasis was on pathology and clinical medicine. Problems soon became apparent, and in 1955, Dr. R. Keith Cannan, chairman of the NRC Division of Medical Sciences, formed a team led by Dr. Thomas Francis, professor of epidemiology at the University of Michigan, to produce an objective, scientific appraisal of the ABCC program. This appraisal resulted in a plan for a long-term epidemiologic study of the survivors. One of the needs identified by the Francis group was collaboration by strong U.S. departments that would assist in recruiting scientists, provide scientific direction, and lend prestige to the program. The Yale and University of California at Los Angeles medical schools agreed to sponsor medical and pathology efforts, respectively, and the Medical Follow-up Agency (MFUA) assumed responsibility for statistics (there was not yet a department of epidemiology at ABCC). For many years, MFUA personnel rotated between Washington and Japan, and helped to recruit statistical staff. Later, an arrangement with the University of Washington greatly strengthened the program.

In 1975, the ABCC was succeeded by the Radiation Effects Research Foundation (RERF). Under the auspices of this organization, epidemiologic research concerning the long-term health outcomes of survivors of the atomic bombings of Hiroshima and Nagasaki, and their descendants, continues today. The association of the MFUA with the studies of the ABCC and subsequently the RERF, although in some ways a distraction from the studies of veterans, was on balance a very positive development. The research in Japan gave MFUA staff a degree of expertise and competence in studying the effects of ionizing radiation. These skills found expression in many other projects, such as studies of veterans who had participated in tests of nuclear weapons.

Selected Reference

Putnam, F. Hiroshima and Nagasaki revisited: The Atomic Bomb Casualty Commission and the Radiation Effects Research Foundation. *Perspectives in Biology and Medicine* 37(4):515–545, 1994.

Japan to assist in the commission's work.[77] Cannan decided that it would be best for the statistical program of the commission if senior statisticians from the Follow-up Agency took successive tours of duty in Japan. He hoped that Beebe would make the first formal tour, beginning in July 1958. When Beebe went to Japan, data from the commission would be sent to Washington, enabling some of the commission's work to be done by the Follow-up Agency staff there. The assignment strained the agency's staff. Perhaps for this reason, the agency, for the very first time, had no formal proposal before the Committee on Veterans Medical Problems when it met in December 1957.[78]

Reflecting at the end of 1957, Beebe noted that study findings often defied expectations. He pointed to the study of psychoneurosis that had been done by Norman Brill, using a sample of 1,500 Army and Navy veterans. Only a few of the men who had broken down could have been identified on induction. Their breakdowns reflected the stresses of war and could not easily be foreseen. Many men with an apparent predisposition to psychoneurosis served with distinction during the war. Upon follow-up, only 8 percent seemed to be severely disabled, and suicide was comparatively rare. These findings could not have been predicted in advance: it took a follow-up study to reveal them. Similarly, the studies of hepatitis and of scrub typhus addressed the question of whether an acute infectious disease set the stage for a chronic, degenerative process. Here too, only empirical research of the sort the agency performed could uncover the answers. Beebe noted also the extent to which the agency relied on statistical epidemiology, rather than clinical follow-up, and the fact that some of the agency's work involved using records from World War I.[79]

As Beebe recognized, the agency's studies followed no orderly pattern. In fiscal year 1957, for example, the agency contemplated studies on rheumatoid arthritis, multiple sclerosis, lesions of the intervertebral disk, infectious hepatitis, and coronary artery disease. In addition, the agency received requests to collaborate with VA hospitals on two clinical trials, one of "chemical adjuvants to surgery in the treatment of cancer" and the other of "anticoagulants and diet in the treatment of cerebrovascular disease." The former series of clinical trials became an ongoing effort for more than two decades. In the same year, the staff assisted in producing an article on a treatment for multiple sclerosis and helped to complete a monograph for the VA on peripheral nerve regeneration.[80]

TRANSITIONS IN PERSONNEL

The late 1950s marked an important transition in the agency's history. For the first time, the title of the agency in some official reports became the Medical Follow-up Agency (MFUA), although references to the Follow-up Agency were also common. Whatever the agency's name, the staff, with the aid of its clinical investigators, managed to complete five studies, including the study of Buerger's disease, in fiscal year 1958.

Changes in personnel also occurred at this time. As expected, Gilbert Beebe took a leave of absence to serve as chief of biostatistics for the Atomic Bomb Casualty Commission. In February 1959, Bernard Cohen suffered a heart attack, and he did not return to work until September 1960. To compensate for this loss, the agency hired two new professional staff members, the most significant additions since Jablon and Cohen had joined the agency a decade before. Dean Nefzger, who had a Ph.D. in psychology and statistics, came to the agency from the University of Buffalo. Robert Keehn left his job as director of the Bureau of Vital Statistics for the State of Connecticut to work for the MFUA.[81]

This transition in personnel slowed the agency's progress. When Gilbert Beebe went to Japan, he had to put aside three manuscripts on subjects related to acute viral hepatitis, cold injuries, and arterial injuries. When Bernard Cohen got sick, it stopped his work on monographs related to Hodgkin's disease and Buerger's disease. Michael DeBakey, Cohen's collaborator on the second study, was overwhelmed with other work and unable to attend to the Medical Follow-up Agency's projects.[82] Then, once Beebe returned to Washington, Jablon left for Japan, a pattern that would be repeated in the years ahead as staff members shuttled back and forth.

In Beebe's absence, the staff concentrated on five major projects during fiscal year 1959. The first involved a follow-up of about 2,200 cases of coronary heart disease that had been diagnosed in the Army during World War II. The second study, which had a similar design, centered on the natural progression of multiple sclerosis in 850 soldiers diagnosed during the war. The third study consisted of the clinical trial of chemotherapy as an adjuvant to surgery in the treatment of cancer, and the fourth was a study of men admitted to Army hospitals during World War II with ulcerative colitis or regional ileitis.[83]

The fifth study, which proved to be the most time-consuming, concerned twins. The agency began the the cross-country search of birth records to obtain the names of live, white, male twins born between 1917 and 1927. During the first year of the project, the agency enlisted the participation of 44 of the 48 (soon to be 50) states and obtained information from 29 states, yielding 45,000 pairs of twin births and 170 sets of all-male triplets. Using the VA Master Index, project staff identified 6,000 pairs of twins who had both joined the military. Simultaneously, work began at the FBI to find the induction fingerprints of eligible twins. Even at this preliminary stage the project went over budget, since there were more twins than investigators had anticipated and the state offices charged more for their services than the investigators had expected.[84] The VA, which financed the project along with the National Institutes of Health, agreed to make up the difference. Additionally, the project began to encounter delays, particularly in the FBI phase of the work. This in turn slowed progress in the next phase of the project—testing the effectiveness of using fingerprints to predict zygosity by comparing fingerprints with clinical observations.[85]

Even as work on the twins and other major projects continued, and despite the absence of key personnel, the agency managed to launch four new studies in fiscal year 1960. One focused on the morbidity and VA compensation experiences of soldiers who developed Japanese encephalitis during service in the Far East. Another looked at the long-term effects of acute infectious hepatitis on soldiers who served in Korea in 1950 and 1951. During treatment of this disease, doctors enforced a vigorous rehabilitation regimen: bed rest was discouraged and rehabilitation measures were started early in the recovery. The study sought to discover whether this course of managing the disease increased long-term complications. A third study followed up on a clinical trial of an influenza vaccine that had been conducted by the Army between 1951 and 1953 to see whether an oil adjuvant vaccine produced excess morbidity or mortality. The fourth study emphasized the agency's statistical expertise and involved an examination of the effectiveness of direct ultraviolet irradiation during surgery in preventing postoperative wound infections. During the year, agency staff published seven articles or monographs in publications such as the *Journal of Neurosurgery*.[86]

DECLINE OF THE COMMITTEE ON VETERANS MEDICAL PROBLEMS

The agency undertook all of this work without much guidance from the Committee on Veterans Medical Problems. William S. Middleton, the VA's chief medical officer, contemplated altering the committee's structure to reflect the fact that the VA no longer had much contract research and sponsored only a few projects conducted by the Medical Follow-up Agency. Keith Cannan of the National Academy of Sciences, for his part, noted the need to support the MFUA with competent advice but questioned the need for a committee such as the CVMP to provide this service.[87]

Gilbert Beebe, who was back from Japan, realized that very little of the agency's work was being done in VA hospitals and that the agency had not influenced the VA's research program. He argued that the "yield of the program might be significantly increased if the committee were able and willing to function more actively in the area of program planning." Still, Beebe found much to applaud. He cited the great variety of projects completed, the warm response the MFUA had received from federal agencies, and the unexpected opportunities for epidemiological investigation. The twin studies, in particular, revealed "an unexpected depth in the veteran material."[88] Above all else, the program had produced a considerable volume of new scientific information.

The Committee on Veterans Medical Problems, for its part, believed that Beebe needed to do more to publicize the agency's program. The Committee suggested that he write an article for a national journal. Keith Cannan said that other NRC committees might be able to help more if they were "reacquainted with the potentialities of the program." DeBakey thought that the agency might broaden its approach to work with nonveteran groups. The follow-up technique was receiving more emphasis in clinical research, and the agency staff might offer its services more widely. Although the agency did not immediately act on DeBakey's suggestion, the question of the breadth of the study population would recur.[89]

Toward the end of 1961, it seemed increasingly likely that the Committee on Veterans Medical Problems would not be reappointed in 1962. Beebe worked to formulate a new committee to advise the follow-up program. He approached a representative of the American Psychiatric Association and told him of the need for a psychiatrist to serve as a member of the new committee. He also talked with his professional associates in the field of epidemiology.[90]

In January 1962, Keith Cannan held an important discussion with the NRC about the future of the Committee on Veterans Medical Problems and the Medical Follow-up Agency. He found the response of the Veterans Administration to the suggestions of the NRC unsatisfactory. The group agreed to let the committee remain on the roster until June 1962, after which time it would be abolished. At the same time, the group decided that the agency should remain with the NRC and that an effort would be made to publicize its value and purpose.[91]

Beebe, Jablon, and Cohen all felt more comfortable with the role of scholar than the role of advocate. During this period, Seymour Jablon published an essay on the characteristics of a clinical trial and was the second author of a piece on acute epidemic hemorrhagic fever. Gilbert Beebe's long report on the possible relation of lung cancer to mustard gas injury (see Box 6) and his study of the 1918 influenza epidemic among World War I veterans appeared in the *Journal of the National Cancer Institute*. While in Japan, Jablon and Dr. A. Earl Walker reviewed their draft monograph on head wounds. Bernard Cohen continued to work with Michael DeBakey on their monograph about Buerger's disease.[92]

Much as he would have preferred to do his own statistical research, Beebe spent a considerable amount of time in 1961 and 1962 trying to present the agency's mission to a larger audience. He wrote an informal history of the program in which he highlighted some of the agency's major accomplishments. Beebe noted that as the program developed, it produced findings of interest to a wide range of doctors. Each study, he suggested, told a scientifically important story.[93]

As the end of the Committee on Veterans Medical Problems drew near, Beebe intensified his search to find people to serve on a new advisory committee. With help from outsiders, Beebe drew up a tentative list of 18 people that included, among others, Michael DeBakey; psychiatrist Alexander Leighton; internist and geneticist (and twin) Victor McKusick; Brian MacMahon, a Harvard epidemiologist interested in chronic disease; and Abraham Lilienfeld, a Johns Hopkins epidemiologist interested in cancer studies.[94]

In July 1962, Keith Cannan let the members of the Committee on Veterans Medical Problems know that the committee would not be reappointed. His first letter was to Michael DeBakey. "It is hard to put into words a measure of our

---

BOX 6
Studies of Lung Cancer Mortality and
Exposure to Mustard Gas

In July 1917, in a field outside of Ypres, Belgium, mustard gas was used for the first time in World War I. In total, mustard gas would cause nearly 400,000 casualties during the war, more than any other chemical agent. One of the long-term effects of exposure to mustard gas is chronic bronchitis, but it was unknown whether the long-term risk of lung cancer would be elevated in men who had been exposed.

Three samples of World War I veterans totaling 7,151 U.S. white males were followed up for mortality through 1956 and again through 1965 in order to learn whether a single exposure to mustard gas with respiratory injury was associated with increased risk of lung cancer in later life.

Men born between 1889 and 1893 who were either (1) exposed to mustard gas as documented by skin burns, or (2) hospitalized with pneumonia in 1918, or (3) hospitalized with wounds of the extremities were traced via the Veterans Administration's death records.

Results of both follow-up studies failed to establish a definite carcinogenic effect for mustard gas, although the studies did find a relative risk of 1.3 for lung cancer mortality in exposed as compared to unexposed men. Observed deaths from lung cancer represented 2.5 percent of the mustard gas group, 1.8 percent of the pneumonia group, and 1.9 percent of unexposed men for the period 1919–1965. Even though these results were equivocal, presumably because men in the study received a relatively light dose, the second follow-up did find evidence suggesting a latency period for a carcinogenic effect ranging from 22 to 37 years.

Although mustard gas was not used in World War II, both sides produced and stockpiled such weapons and prepared for their possible use. As part of this preparation, roughly 4,000 servicemen participated as experimental subjects in tests of the short-term effects of mustard gas. However, there has been no follow-up assessment of the long-term health effects of mustard gas exposure among these subjects.

Selected References

Beebe, G.W. Lung cancer in World War I veterans: Possible relation to mustard-gas injury and 1918 influenza epidemic. *Journal of the National Cancer Institute* 25:1231–1251, 1960.

Norman, J.E. Lung cancer mortality in World War I veterans with mustard-gas injury: 1919–1965. *Journal of the National Cancer Institute* 54:311–317, 1975.

---

indebtedness to you over so many years and in such a diversity of problems," he wrote. Writing to William Stone, then chair of the committee, Cannan noted, "We plan to continue the program of medical follow-up studies and will need the active guidance of a group of medical investigators." He added, however, that he had not decided on the composition or the exact mission of such a group. Esmond Long, a long-time committee member, said that the fact that the follow-up program would continue was "reassuring." Don Mainland, the New York University medical statistician who had evaluated the committee, agreed that the follow-up program still had what he called "potentialities, but I would think that its future would not be easy to plan."[95] Ultimately, Cannan delayed the appointment of the successor committee for several years, allowing the agency to operate on the advice of ad hoc groups as it worked out various problems related to its future.

There were two problems as the CVMP passed into memory. First, the Veterans Administration had funded the Committee on Veterans Medical Problems and no similar means of support existed for a committee that would advise the Medical Follow-up Agency. As Cannan put it, the agency had to be supported on a "fluid basis," and the NRC was actively pursuing this possibility with the National Institutes of Health. Second, the MFUA was a "research tool, not a research institution." It therefore needed to develop "a better relationship with clinical investigation."[96]

The death of Bernard Cohen in 1963 exacerbated this second problem. For 15 years he had played a key role in the program's development. At the time of his death, his monograph with Michael DeBakey on Buerger's disease was in press, and he had completed major papers on coronary heart disease and Hodgkin's disease. He also played a key role in the twin project. Adding to the interruption caused by Cohen's death, the agency continued its relationship with the Atomic Bomb Casualty Commission. Dean Nefzger left in 1962 for a two-year tour of duty, and Robert Keehn planned to go to Japan in 1963.

Simply put, the agency faced a desperate need for new staff to deal with a growing workload. For the twin study, it hired Glenn Atkinson, a graduate student in statistics at Cornell with considerable background in biology. He spent his first few months with the agency at the University of Michigan, studying human genetics with Dr. Neel. After a brief tenure with the agency, however, he left in 1965. In December 1962, Zdenek Hrubec joined the agency after having spent three years working for the ABCC in Nagasaki. He held a doctorate in public health statistics from the School of Public Health at Pittsburgh. Unlike Atkinson, Hrubec remained with the agency for a lengthy period of time and ultimately became the lead staff officer for the twin study.

The new staff members went to work on projects with subjects as disparate as multiple sclerosis (see Box 7) and herniated lumbar disks. Only one of the studies, on the effects of light mineral oil used as an adjuvant in experimental trials of influenza vaccines, was completed by fiscal year 1964. Even so, the agency initiated two new studies: one a long-term follow-up of x-ray technicians trained by the Army in World War II and the other an examination of the association between late-appearing cataracts and exposure to military radar. As these studies proceeded, Beebe and his associates also tried to shore up the statistical resources available to the agency. They persuaded the VA to retain a representative sample (2 percent) of the World War II National Service Life Insurance record cards, an invaluable source for developing control groups.[97]

BOX 7
Studies of Multiple Sclerosis

One of the most prolific subjects of study for the Medical Follow-up Agency has been the study of multiple sclerosis (MS). Beginning in 1963, MFUA staff and collaborators began a series of publications on the natural history of MS based on a set of cases identified from World War II Army hospitalization records. Papers were published on the progression from optic neuropathy to multiple sclerosis, the onset bout and its clinical features, long-term survival, clinical and laboratory findings at first diagnosis, and correlates of clinical change.

Partly as a result of these investigations, it was decided to attempt to assemble a much larger series of MS cases and controls from military sources so that topics such as geographic variation in MS risk could be studied. With the assistance of collaborators, MFUA assembled a set of 5,300 MS cases and matched controls who served in World War II and the Korean War, and embarked on a long series of reports based on this material. The report on race, sex, and geography, for example, showed that white females had the highest risk of multiple sclerosis, followed by white males and then black males. The risk of multiple sclerosis was shown to increase substantially by geographic location, with veterans who were born or entered military service at more northern locations having a higher risk of developing MS. This increase in MS risk with latitude was shown not to be due to climatic factors, and migrants who moved south (e.g., those who were born in the North and entered service in the South) showed a substantially reduced risk of multiple sclerosis, whereas those who moved north from the middle tier of the United States had a substantially increased risk of MS. Subsequent research showed that age at onset of MS is younger as one moves northward.

Using aggregate data from the U.S. Census, it was shown that MS risk was significantly higher in states whose residents reported higher rates of Swedish or Scandinavian ancestry; English and Dutch ancestry were associated with lower risk of multiple sclerosis. However, when ethnicity was determined for each individual by using the surname, there was no association of ethnicity with MS risk, except possibly for southern European ancestry. An analysis of other risk factors

---

NEW CORE FUNDS

In fiscal year 1964, the agency's efforts at outreach and modernization appeared to be producing results. The National Institutes of Health joined the VA and the Department of Defense in providing general support, as distinguished from specific project support. In addition to the "research resources" contract, the NIH also awarded the agency a contract for its twin study. The new core funds, beginning in fiscal year 1965, made it possible for the agency to engage in more planning, undertake more pilot studies, and maintain the data bases on which its work depended. At the same time, the agency received new computers for its work, a move that made its data processing easier and enabled it to work more effectively with the Veterans Administration.[98]

With more funds and better hardware in place, the agency and the NRC turned once again to the task of appointing an advisory committee. In constructin white males showed that in addition to northern latitude, higher levels of education, an urban versus rural address, poor uncorrected visual acuity at entry into service, and a high proportion of persons with Swedish ancestry in the state from which a subject entered the military all increased the risk of MS.

As the MFUA begins its second half-century, research on the topic of multiple sclerosis continues. Mortality follow-up studies of the two case series described above are under way, as is the assembly of a post-Korean War series of matched MS cases and controls.

Selected References

Beebe, G.W., Kurtzke, J.F., Nagler, B., Nefzger, M.D., Auth, T.L., Kurland, L.T. Studies on the natural history of multiple sclerosis. V. Long-term survival in young men. *Archives of Neurology* 22:215–225, 1970.

Kurtzke, J.F., Beebe, G.W., Nagler, B., Auth, T.L., Kurland, L.T., Nefzger, M.D. Studies on the natural history of multiple sclerosis. III. Epidemiologic analysis of the Army experience of World War II. *Neurology* 17:1–17, 1967.

Kurtzke, J.F., Beebe, G.W., Norman, J.E., Jr. Epidemiology of multiple sclerosis in U.S. veterans. I: Race, sex, and geographic distribution. *Neurology* 29(Sept.): 1228–1235, 1979.

Kurtzke, J.F., Beebe, G.W., Norman, J.E., Jr. Epidemiology of multiple sclerosis in U.S. veterans. III: Migration and the risk of MS. *Neurology* 35(5):672–678, 1985.

Kurtzke, J.F., Page, W.F. Epidemiology of multiple sclerosis in US veterans. VII. Risk factors for MS. *Neurology* 48(1):204–213, 1997.

Norman, J.E., Jr., Kurtzke, J.F., Beebe, G.W. Epidemiology of multiple sclerosis in U.S. veterans. II. Latitude, climate, and the risk of multiple sclerosis. *Journal of Chronic Disease* 36:551–559, 565–567, 1983.

Page, W.F., Mack, T.M., Kurtzke, J.F., Murphy, F.M., Norman, J.E., Jr. Epidemiology of multiple sclerosis in U.S. veterans. VI. Population ancestry and surname ethnicity as risk factors for multiple sclerosis. *Neuroepidemiology* 14:286–296, 1995.

ing this committee, Beebe thought it important to find people who had a demonstrated interest in the natural history of disease; a knowledge of the medical bureaucracies of the armed forces or the VA; broad medical interests; and specific competence in internal medicine, general surgery, epidemiology, psychiatry, pathology, medical statistics, or medical genetics. He also wanted to appoint people who had at least some knowledge of the follow-up program. He divided his list of possible nominees among epidemiologists, public health statisticians, and other medical specialists. He favored an epidemiologist, such as Thomas Francis or Abraham Lilienfeld, as chair. Francis had the added benefit of already serving on the Advisory Committee for the Atomic Bomb Casualty Commission. Beebe also hoped that the NRC would appoint a small subcommittee to supervise the twin study, perhaps chaired by James Neel.[99] On December 16, 1964, Cannan wrote Thomas Francis at the University of Michigan and asked him to accept the chairmanship of the advisory committee. He noted that the NRC had delayed appointing the group until it learned about the application to the NIH for a research facility support grant. With the award of the grant, "we now have much more opportunity to develop a balanced program in a more orderly way than in the days when support came, in the main, from project grants."[100]

After Francis declined the committee chairmanship, Cannan turned to Dr. Brian MacMahon, professor in Harvard's Department of Epidemiology in the School of Public Health. Cannan urged MacMahon to form "a group of active individuals, largely investigators, who would be interested in directing the program into the most promising areas of research in the natural history of disease."[101] MacMahon, whose experience with the MFUA had left him with "a deep respect for its professional staff, and also with considerable enthusiasm about the potential of its research program," agreed to head the new oversight body. This began a relationship that lasted for more than three decades.[102]

COMMITTEE ON EPIDEMIOLOGY AND VETERANS FOLLOW-UP STUDIES

The very name of the new Committee on Epidemiology and Veterans Follow-up Studies (CEVFUS) reflected "the increased evidence of potential for epidemiologic as well as other studies on the natural history of disease."[103] Charging the committee to "develop the scientific content of the program and to oversee the work of the Follow-up Agency and collaborating investigators," Cannan wrote to one committee member that he expected the committee "to be involved in a constant reassessment and reformulation of program in response to the progress of medical research generally."[104] The committee contained some carryovers from the former CVMP, including DeBakey, and included a rich mix of epidemiologists, public health professionals, and statisticians from academia and the public sector. Public health figures outnumbered clinicians. Other than DeBakey, the clinicians included Dr. William S. Jordan, professor of internal medicine at the University of Virginia, and Dr. Louis J. Zeldis, professor of pathology at the University of California School of Medicine. Among others, Dr. Frederick H. Epstein, professor of epidemiology in the University of Michigan's School of Public Health, brought expertise in epidemiology to the committee.[105]

Taking stock of its mission as the new committee got organized, the Medical Follow-up Agency could note that the "medical research environment" was "much more favorable for a program that is population-based and in which statistical methods play a primary role" than had been the case at the agency's founding in 1946. In the interim, the MFUA had "succeeded in forging a practical tool of wide applicability and demonstrated effectiveness," despite the limitations inherent in data sets specific to the military veteran population. With funding and organizational improvements in place, studies flourished and the MFUA entered a new era.[106]

If statistics were to be the agency's primary focus, then attention needed to be paid to the tools of statistical analysis. In this regard, Seymour Jablon made efforts to integrate the National Academy of Science's (NAS's) IBM 1440 mainframe computer into the MFUA's procedures (see photo), work that necessitated hiring new personnel and training ongoing staff, transferring various card files to computer tape, and developing new agency procedures. Jablon emphasized the development of "utility" programs that could be applied easily to specific problems as they arose. This would reduce the need for time-consuming programming. In all, the new computer would allow the agency to bring to "more refined, more elaborate, and deeper forms of analysis" to bear on the data sets at the heart of the agency's procedures.[107]

THE NEW COMMITTEE'S MISSION

The Committee on Epidemiology and Veterans Follow-up Studies met for the first time on November 26, 1965. Dr. MacMahon described the committee's

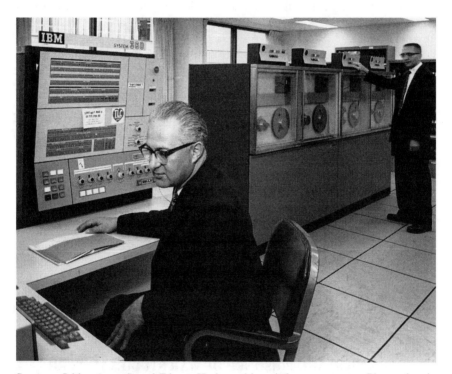

Seymour Jablon (seated) and Zdenec Hrubec with mainframe computer. Photo taken in the Joseph Henry Building, Data Processing Center, winter of 1967–1968. Photo courtesy of the National Academy of Sciences Archives.

mission as a combination of advisory, stimulative, and protective functions, to "bridge the gap between the program and the investigator that derived from the composition of the Follow-up Agency and its location" in the NAS. Following a discussion of the methods and resources of the agency, the committee heard a summary of the studies in progress. Research efforts were being directed at heart disease, multiple sclerosis, and the consequences of occupational exposure to ionizing radiation.

Ongoing efforts in fiscal year 1965 included the study of long-term survival in Hodgkin's disease, the long-term follow-up of testicular tumors, the natural history of multiple sclerosis, and the follow-up of more than a thousand World War II veterans diagnosed with herniated lumbar disks (the agency's only clinical project then in operation). Agency staff noted that "two or three projects usually terminate each year," leaving room for "two or three" new projects each fiscal year, figures that would remain fairly consistent for the next decade. In 1965, planning began on at least five new studies: the possible influence of blood type on the incidence of salivary cancers, the link between early incidence of heat stroke and heat exhaustion and later-in-life heart and circulatory disease, the causes of chronic kidney diseases and disorders, a pilot study of amyotrophic lateral sclerosis (also known as Lou Gehrig's disease), and the treatment of thyroid nodules.[108]

At its second meeting, in early 1966, the committee began the task of agency oversight. MFUA staff described an important trend in the program, the shift from clinical follow-up studies to epidemiologic studies. This trend accentuated the emphasis on record studies at the expense of clinical examinations. Similarly, studies of mortality (as opposed to morbidity) became more frequent as the World War II cohort continued to age. Even in studies of morbidity, the distance from military service made it more difficult to locate some of the men.[109]

The agency's program development had suffered during its financial uncertainty in the early 1960s. In the meantime, agency staff had focused on ongoing efforts, such as the study of the epidemiology of multiple sclerosis. This study proved especially fruitful in 1966 and produced a paper given at the American Academy of Neurology, as well as publications in both domestic and international neurological journals. MFUA researchers found geographic variation in preservice environment, as well as more important differences associated with urbanization, socioeconomic status, and race, to be significant variables in identifying veterans with multiple sclerosis. Other ongoing projects included studies of the epidemiology of coronary heart disease, the Hodgkin's disease project, and the study of occupational exposure to x-rays.[110]

THE TWIN AND PRISONER OF WAR STUDIES MATURE

One of the most important ongoing projects in 1966 was the study of prisoners of war (POWs) (see Box 8), an effort to follow the experience of World War

II and Korean War POWs with respect to both mortality and morbidity. A resurvey of the former POWs began in March 1965. This study provided investigators with an unwelcome reminder of the ephemerality of paper records when, in 1965, an entire carton of records was discarded as trash by the night janitorial staff of the MFUA's downtown Washington office. After more than two days of excavation efforts at the Fairfax Sanitary Land Fill in Virginia, Beebe's staff gave up the search. Soldiering on, the agency continued the study throughout the mid-1960s, sending a mail questionnaire to its cohort of 2,500 POWs. The questions in the mailing, targeted to determine mental adjustment as well as physical well-being, were compared with those of an equal number of combat veterans who had not been captured.[111]

In a 1967 letter from staff statistician M. Dean Nefzger to Gilbert Beebe (in Japan on his rotation for the Atomic Bomb Casualty Commission), Nefzger noted that work on the POW study was "proceeding apace." The data had been collected, the index work completed, the mortality information coded, and the questionnaires analyzed. However, response rates for the questionnaires remained relatively low, around 70 percent, in part because of questions of the confidentiality of key information that was required from the Internal Revenue Service and the Social Security Administration. Problems with these agencies were endemic for the rest of the decade, suggesting the limits of the low-profile agency's ability to cut through Great Society-era red tape. Nefzger and those who followed him on the project turned increasingly to private organizations for help with the crucial matter of locating veterans who had lost contact with the Veterans Administration or who refused to respond to questionnaires.[112]

By offering the use of their mailing lists to the agency for name and address comparison and by frequent mention of its activities in their regular newsletters, veterans organizations proved of great assistance in helping the MFUA locate people in the sample of whom the VA had lost track. However, these organizations also gave the POW study an emotionally charged atmosphere, perhaps not well suited to the scientific method. For example, the American Defenders of Bataan and Corregidor wrote angrily to CEVFUS Chairman MacMahon to inquire why so few members of its organization had been targeted by the MFUA's series of surveys. Seymour Jablon responded for Dr. MacMahon, explaining the concept of "targeted surveys," which would approach only a statistically significant percentage of the entire World War II POW cohort. Still, the MFUA's relationship with this and other veterans organizations remained problematic. In general, learning how to deal with the emotional and political responses to its studies became increasingly important for the agency. By 1969, Gilbert Beebe was noting in correspondence that the POW study was "controversial at the level of federal legislation and VA policy, and any data that we generate are very likely to be used, even abused."[113]

The MFUA's study of 16,000 veteran twins, another long-term study, gained momentum in the mid-1960s. At first it suffered from the death of study director

---

BOX 8
Morbidity Studies of Former Prisoners of War

For nearly its entire history, the Medical Follow-up Agency has been conducting mortality (see Box 2) and morbidity studies of former prisoners of war (POWs). Although the original POW study dealt in part with morbidity, the third study in the series, published in 1975, was the first major study devoted solely to POW morbidity. It is still arguably the best single study of the health of American former prisoners of war. In this extensive article, it was reported that the most persistent sequelae of military captivity were psychiatric, manifested in higher hospitalization rates and VA disability awards. These patterns were seen in all groups of former POWs, although they were more severe among those from the Pacific theater in World War II and from the Korean War. Excess morbidity was also found to correlate well with retrospective accounts of weight loss, nutritional deficiencies, and symptoms during captivity.

Data collection for the fifth study in the POW series took place during 1984–1985. Depressive symptoms were assessed using the Center for Epidemiologic Studies Depression scale (CES-D). The study found a three- to fivefold excess in depressive symptoms among former POWs nearly 40 years after repatriation and also found that greater depression could be linked to self-reported weight loss and harshness of treatment during captivity. A number of reports have been prepared that link current depressive symptomatology with various factors. For example, it was shown that being younger and having less education at the time of capture, experiencing more medical symptoms during captivity, and receiving less social support after release were generally predictive of increased long-term psychiatric maladjustment.

Dr. Bernard Cohen and the fact that Seymour Jablon found verifying the zygosity of the twins more difficult than expected. His rotation in Japan with the ABCC for three years at a key moment in the planning process made finding computer time to run the necessary trials difficult and further slowed the process. The FBI continued to obstruct release of the remainder of the requested fingerprints for the twins cohort to the MFUA. When Jablon returned to the states and finished his computer trials, his findings were not as conclusive as he had hoped. Nonetheless, he and Professor Neel, the principal investigator on the project from the University of Michigan's Department of Human Genetics, determined that a combination of fingerprint analysis, serological testing, and, most especially, questionnaire analysis was sufficient to make the necessary determinations for formation of the NAS–NRC Twins Registry. They co-authored a paper that announced the Twins Registry to the medical world and interested a large number of investigators.[114]

Having anticipated this interest, Jablon and Neel brought the matter to CEVFUS in its March 1966 meeting. The committee agreed that the twins had to

In 1996, a book-length report of the sixth study in the series was published. This study involved the first attempted clinical follow-up examination survey of former prisoners of war. For this study, former POWs and comparison individuals were invited to be examined at a nearby VA hospital by local clinicians. Unfortunately, relatively few POWs and even fewer comparisons chose to be examined, which limited the value of the data collected. Nevertheless, analysis of the examination data yielded a number of medical findings of potential interest and again confirmed the high rate of psychiatric illness among POWs. Posttraumatic stress disorder (PTSD) was studied for the first time (the diagnostic category did not exist officially at the time the studies began) and was found to have occurred at especially high rates in former POWs. Subsequent reports have also been prepared on PTSD and on stroke among former POWs.

Selected References

Beebe, G.W. Follow-up studies of World War II and Korean War prisoners. II. Morbidity, disability, and maladjustments. *American Journal of Epidemiology* 101:400–422, 1975.

Page, W.F. *The Health of Former Prisoners of War: Results for the Medical Examination Survey of Former POWs of World War II and the Korean Conflict.* Washington, D.C.: National Academy Press, 1992.

Page, W.F., Ostfeld, A.M. Malnutrition and subsequent ischemic heart disease in former prisoners of war of World War II and the Korean conflict. *Journal of Clinical Epidemiology* 47:1437–1441, 1994.

Page, W.F., Engdahl, B.E., Eberly, R.B. Prevalence and correlates of depressive symptoms among former prisoners of war. *Journal of Nervous and Mental Disease* 179(11):670–677, 1991.

be guarded from overzealous investigators who might abuse their good will, that the MFUA should regularly update the mortality and morbidity of the panel, and that further efforts should be made to seek fingerprint information from the FBI in order to ascertain zygosity definitively. The latter effort, however, never reached fruition, even with new leadership at the FBI. In addition, efforts began in 1966 to make the previously ad hoc subcommittee on twins a permanent fixture of the CEVFUS–MFUA structure.[115]

From its earliest days, CEVFUS functioned as far more than a rubber stamp; instead it took a hard look at the methods and appropriateness of all studies submitted. The committee considered the first three proposals to use the NAS–NRC Twins Registry in 1967. One, which became an ongoing study with follow-up into the 1980s, compared smoking patterns and other potential risk factors with the incidence of lung cancer and aimed to demonstrate the disparate roles that heredity and environmental factors played in these diseases. The other two proposals, however, lacked sufficient justification for tying them into the Twins Registry per se, and so the committee rejected them. Dr. Neel estimated that although "12 to 15 really good studies" might come out of the registry, making "the whole effort of creating" it worthwhile, a much larger number of applications would have to be sifted through in order to find these good applications. Throughout the late 1960s, Dr. Neel continued to push for a "hard-nosed" approach in order to weed out those studies that did not have a "real appreciation of the nuances" or "limitations" of the twins approach.[116]

Early studies of twins were evenly divided between those that required clinical examination of the veteran twins and epidemiological studies that were used to judge the heritability of a particular disease. Over time, the clinical follow-up studies became less common, in part because of the cost and management issues involved in getting men to submit to examination and in ensuring consistency in examination procedures among doctors. Typically, twin studies measured concordance for a disease between both members of a twin pair and then compared these results for monozygotic and dizygotic twins. Theoretically, this method allowed a researcher to determine the degree to which the disease in question was a product of genetic instead of environmental factors. Neel, Hrubec, and the other twin study managers recognized the limitations of such research, however. Twin brothers would likely have shared environmental exposures, for example, and the twin studies were inherently observational rather than experimental. Moreover, since the presence of a particular disease in individual members of the cohort would change over time, the file necessarily had to be followed up over time, incurring additional future costs. Despite these limitations, however, the MFUA twin cohort (see Box 9) became a key resource in epidemiologic and heritability studies for several decades.[117]

From the beginning, CEVFUS members, especially James Neel, expressed concern that the Twin Registry would attract researchers with poorly designed studies that ran the risk of violating the confidentiality of the twins or exhausting their patience (e.g., by following up too often or overusing a regional cohort that had been used recently for another study). The committee feared in particular that a single region-specific study might exhaust the region's twin population for the foreseeable future. A possible solution was for researchers to combine forces in a collaborative effort, but this would be impossible in the case of clinical follow-up where a number of the examinations had already been conducted.

Then there was the problem of keeping the twins interested. CEVFUS urged the agency to feed the data back to the twins "to help maintain their interest." Unfortunately, despite sporadic efforts, this feedback plan proved too unwieldy, particularly in the largest studies, leaving the twins unaware of the uses to which their responses had been put. Occasionally, they would write angry letters to the MFUA staff, demanding to know what the agency was doing with their information.[118]

BOX 9
The NAS–NRC Twin Registry

Since the time of Sir Francis Galton, studies of human twins have provided material with which to study the relative effects of genetics and environment. When identical twins are more similar with respect to some characteristic than fraternal twins, this is taken as evidence of a genetic influence on a particular characteristic. In 1958, the Medical Follow-up Agency began a project to identify white male twins who had jointly entered military service during World War II, an effort funded by the National Institutes of Health and the Veterans Administration. Beginning with birth records provided by 42 vital statistics offices, 108,000 searches were made by hand against VA files to determine veteran status. In the end, nearly 16,000 twin pairs were identified in which both members had served in the military.

Certain baseline data were abstracted from VA and military records, an initial questionnaire was mailed to the twin pairs, and anthropometric and fingerprint data were used to determine zygosity (i.e., to differentiate identical from fraternal twins). Interestingly, the single best question for determining zygosity by self-report—As children, were you and your twin as alike as two peas in a pod?—is essentially a translation of a similar item used in the Danish and Swedish twin registries and accurately predicts zygosity roughly 95 percent of the time. Subsequent follow-up data have come primarily from computerized VA records and mail surveys. A subset of roughly 500 twin pairs, the National Heart, Lung, and Blood Institute twins, have been examined by investigators four different times at clinical centers around the country.

More than 200 journal articles have made use of the Twin Registry. Published articles cover a variety of topics. Among these are articles on smoking and respiratory function, schizophrenia, heart disease, bone mass, eye disease, type A behavior, blood chemistry profiles, headache, blood pressure, personality traits, financial earnings, dietary intake, fingerprint patterns, weight change and body fat distribution, alcoholism, cancer, diabetes, antisocial behavior, Alzheimer's disease, alcohol and tobacco consumption, suicide, declines in cognitive functioning, and prostate disease.

Selected References

Hrubec, Z., Neel, J.V. The National Academy of Sciences–National Research Council Twin Registry: Ten years of operation. in W.E. Nance, ed., *Twin Research. Proceedings of the Second International Congress on Twin Studies. Part B: Biology and Epidemiology, Progress in Clinical and Biological Research,* Volume 24B. New York: Alan R. Liss, Inc., 1978. Pp. 153–172

Jablon, S., Neel, J.V., Gershowitz, H., Atkinson, G.F. The NAS–NRC Twin Panel: Methods of construction of the panel, zygosity diagnosis, and proposed uses. *American Journal of Human Genetics* 19(March):133–161, 1967.

Page, W.F. Annotation: The National Academy of Sciences–National Research Council Twin Registry. *American Journal of Public Health* 85:617–618, 1995.

THE AGENCY IN THE AGE OF THE GREAT SOCIETY
AND ITS AFTERMATH

In the late 1960s, MFUA staff began to raise concerns about the longevity of the raw material for their studies, particularly the hospital admission punch cards from World War II. As the basis for most of the agency's studies, these punch cards had to be protected against deterioration or, worse, loss, as had been the case with similar Navy admission cards a decade earlier. MFUA estimated the cost of transferring the fragile cards to more permanent magnetic tape in the tens of thousands of dollars, much more than the agency had at its disposal. Forced to look for outside funding, the agency secured money from the National Cancer Institute in fiscal year 1969 and stored the entire series on tape as a basic resource for future studies.[119]

Even as its materials aged, the Medical Follow-up Agency, now staffed by 31 persons (5 professionals, 26 support staff) and with an annual budget of more than a half million dollars, reached important milestones in a number of its ongoing studies in 1967. The VA-funded series of controlled therapeutic trials of chemotherapy in conjunction with cancer surgery reached its tenth year in 1967. In addition to providing authoritative evaluations of the various adjuvant cancer agents tested to improve cancer-free survival after surgery, these trials provided important follow-up data on cancer survival as related to patient characteristics and treatment. Also in the same year, the agency finished a mortality study of patients who had undergone "curative" lung resection for bronchial cancer. The clinical examinations of men with herniated lumbar disks were completed in this year as well, and the agency began an epidemiologic study on the same condition to determine the significance of such variables as tissue degeneration, metabolic disorders, chronic stress, and occupational factors in mortality outcomes. Other ongoing studies during 1967 included an examination of viral and other factors in the etiology of cancer, a cooperative study of lower-limb amputations that aimed to elucidate factors of importance in the rehabilitation process for amputees, and a study of the possible relation of cholesterol levels in the blood to cerebrovascular disease.[120]

Despite this evidence of scientific progress, funding again became an issue for the Medical Follow-up Agency in the late 1960s. Its core support came under attack from within the National Institutes of Health. In part, this attack reflected changing circumstances: Keith Cannan, who had been so instrumental in obtaining funding from the National Institutes of Health, no longer headed the agency's parent Division of Medical Sciences, and NIH staffers with short institutional memories no longer remembered just why they were funding the MFUA. Moreover, NIH faced its own internal budgetary problems. In this, NIH was not alone; the postwar prosperity that had funded the massive expansion of government at all levels was beginning to falter. First the Vietnam War, and later the economic difficulties of the 1970s, meant shrinkage rather than growth for federal agencies concerned with domestic policy.

As a result, the MFUA's application for renewal of the core funding grant from NIH was initially denied after a site visit in October 1967. Following protests, including those of CEVFUS Chairman MacMahon that withdrawal of support would have "tragic" consequences for "the most important single epidemiologic research program in the United States at the present time," NIH agreed to re-fund the agency's programs (including the Twin Registry), but at a lower level than requested. Furthermore, NIH guaranteed funds for only one year. Therefore, although the NIH decision solved the immediate problem, it placed MFUA on shaky financial ground. In the future, NIH would consider requests from the agency only on a year-by-year basis and only on the basis of grants, not core support. Without the assurance of core support for its program, the MFUA faced periodic difficulties throughout the 1970s and especially the 1980s.[121]

In the context of lost core support, individual projects took on a greater importance for the survival of the MFUA. In fiscal year 1968, several projects reached maturity. One was a study of survival rates following "curative" surgery for carcinoma of the colon, as part of the ongoing adjuvant cancer trials. Although none of the drugs tested in these trials was proven to increase survival rates, the trials gave the MFUA significant data for specific studies, one of which found that almost half of the patients studied were still living five years after their colon surgery. Another study considered the possibility of a link between smoking and lower risk of Parkinson's disease, the results of which clearly required further study. Hearing of these results, Dr. Chester S. Keefer of the American College of Physicians called the MFUA's projects "among the most valuable and the most exciting in medicine, [and] among the most important studies that have been made by any group in the NRC . . . very important to the doctor and very important to the family."[122]

In this period the MFUA engaged in an almost bewildering array of studies. Ongoing projects as of late fall 1969 included the study of air pollution and smoking in relation to cardiovascular and respiratory symptoms, as well as a study of schizophrenia that contained a substudy investigating drug-induced parkinsonism in twins with schizophrenia. Other ongoing projects featured an investigation of changes in ocular pressure following application of steroids and a region-based study involving cardiovascular examinations of twins in New England.

In 1969, the Subcommittee on Twin Studies was formally created as an official subunit of the larger committee, with subcommittee membership drawn from CEVFUS as well as external investigators in genetics. In its first meeting, the subcommittee discussed a small number of new proposals and referred the most promising ones to the parent committee, a method of operation that continues to the present day. Beebe privately commended the Twin Registry for offering the MFUA the opportunity to return to the psychiatric studies that had been an early emphasis but had "faded out in the 50's."[123]

In this period as well, the agency continued such projects as the long-term follow-up of men with lumbar disk lesions in World War II, the therapeutic trials of adjuvants to surgical resection in the treatment of cancer, and the study of the natural history of multiple sclerosis. Corroborating a detailed clinical study from 1947 to 1951, an analysis of the possible association between viral hepatitis and subsequent cirrhosis of the liver failed to find a correlation in a mortality follow-up of more than 5,000 Army veterans with viral hepatitis in World War II. Preliminary results from a broad examination of blood type in relation to occlusive and hemorrhagic disease showed that a sample of 816 World War II veterans with records of myocardial infarction had blood type O less frequently than was statistically predicted.[124]

Despite these varied activities, the agency's financial solvency was far from assured. The threat of impending financial hardship led some committee members to suggest that the Atomic Energy Commission (AEC) "should participate in the general institutional support of the MFUA as compensation for its continuing contribution to the ABCC statistical program." Although the AEC arrangement included salary for staff and expenses for their rotations in Japan, committee members argued that the staff exchange was placing a financial burden on the agency that required compensation. Ultimately, nothing came of this matter, in part because Beebe publicly denied that the arrangement in any way weakened the MFUA's program. Still, the very suggestion demonstrated the committee's understanding of both MFUA's financial stringency and the strains that the ABCC rotations placed on the continuity of personnel in the follow-up program. By 1970, the Medical Follow-up Agency staff had dedicated 15 "man-years" to the ABCC rotation.[125]

Although few new studies were added in 1970, significant progress was made in ongoing studies. However, Beebe faced a difficult situation with the resignation of Dean Nefzger in February to take a position with the Johns Hopkins School of Hygiene and Public Health. Efforts to find a qualified replacement took a surprisingly long time, and some projects suffered from the delay of transition, although Nefzger offered to manage several of them temporarily from his new workplace.

In the meantime, work continued on the agency's disparate ongoing projects. Preliminary results for a mortality follow-up of 10,000 inductees discharged from the Army in 1944 for psychoneurosis showed that mortality risk was greater for those who had been diagnosed with psychoneurosis than for the control group. Agency staff presented a paper on regional differences in mortality from cerebrovascular diseases at a conference on stroke epidemiology and began planning for a third test of the completeness of VA information on the mortality of the general population of war veterans. Planning efforts started on a study of behavior patterns in coronary heart disease; an examination of bleeding as a potential side effect of anticoagulant therapy; and an investigation of parental radiation exposure and Down's syndrome, with particular attention to ionizing radiation and radar.[126]

VIETNAM AND THE VETERANS ADMINISTRATION

Although work had settled into a routine, the MFUA faced a changing environment. As the decade reached a close, agency staff found themselves increasingly concerned with how to utilize the Vietnam War experience in future studies, at first purely to strengthen ties with the military establishment. Early response from the military was quite favorable: one Navy Department staffer noted that "a potential gold mine of unique and valuable long-term follow-up medical data" existed regarding various studies conducted in Vietnam, including head injury, shock, and tissue graft studies, along with a variety of neuropsychiatric possibilities. In May 1969, military liaison officers participated in a wide-ranging discussion of the impact of the Vietnam War on the MFUA's future agenda. These liaison officers expressed continued interest in the MFUA and its work.

These same officers noted the limited extent of current procedures for the central indexing of potentially valuable research materials, which inhibited the potential for following up the Vietnam cohort.[127] The MFUA offered to access and preserve specialized rosters that might otherwise become lost or destroyed and to inventory research ideas and investigative interests brought to it. Beebe described the agency's potential research uses of the Vietnam experience as "essentially parasitic," in the sense that the agency would attach itself to already existing data sets and rosters. Ultimately, however, little came of this offer. Nor did the MFUA express much interest in Dr. Lyndon Lee's suggestion that the agency begin to plan to expand the ongoing POW effort to the Vietnam cohort, in part because of the departure of Dr. Dean Nefzger. Ultimately, the military itself took over the effort, in conjunction with the VA and associated outside consultants.[128]

The new chairman of the division of medical sciences, Charles Dunham, who took over in the fall of 1967, wrote to the surgeons general of each service asking that "medical officers be alerted to the research potential of routine medical and allied observations during wartime" and that efforts be made to preserve access in later years to observations made by medical officers in Vietnam. Later, MFUA staff became convinced that these alerts were never distributed by the surgeons general to field officers. However, a series of meetings resulted between MFUA staff and armed forces and VA medical personnel to discuss follow-up studies coming from the war in Vietnam.[129]

The group agreed to consider the need for follow-up studies on battle casualties from the Vietnam War as a test case for a more organized effort to identify priority problems and potential investigators. By late 1970, however, Dr. Beebe was privately concerned that the MFUA was missing an opportunity. "These efforts," he wrote of the meeting with the VA and the military, "have produced little thusfar and raise some basic questions about the feasibility of any real forward planning" of the MFUA's Vietnam War program.[130]

At the third meeting of the ad hoc group on Vietnam issues, the group agreed on a list of ten likely areas of study and picked one, liver injuries, as a "sure-fire subject" around which discussions of program and method would coalesce. Beebe's concerns continued; he wrote Michael DeBakey in the spring of 1971 that "The [Vietnam] effort thusfar has been unsuccessful, but [I] am uncertain why. The meetings have been lacking in inspiration, and participants have not set one another off. The military representatives want to be cooperative, but all are busy and few . . . would themselves be prepared to devote time to such studies. Perhaps it is the enthusiasm of the interested investigator that has been lacking, the compelling zeal of the man who wants to find the answer."[131]

In other words, the military of the 1960s contained no Michael DeBakey, no figure who combined clinical practice and organizational vision in a way that rose above the immediate concerns of the military bureaucracy. Beebe was understandably puzzled; the Medical Follow-up Agency had been founded almost three decades earlier because of "the enthusiasm of the interested investigator" that overflowed in the military medical establishment after World War II. This was a very different war—one that, instead of unifying the nation, divided it, and from which many of the "best and brightest" fled in horror and disgust. Beebe could not mobilize the surgeons general or their top advisers as DeBakey and he had done in the late 1940s. Too many doctors remained outside, evading or even assailing the war effort. Beebe worried that "an aging organization" would begin to falter without the new ideas and fresh outlook of the generation of the 1960s, noting that committee members had "not had much to say about problems growing out of Vietnam."[132]

The liver study gradually came to an end, and, despite some continuing efforts to bring the Vietnam War cohort into the MFUA program of studies, the agency returned its focus to the generation that had served in the 1940s. In 1973, Beebe would write to one CEVFUS member to express his regret that "we have not been able to get any work going on surgical problems growing out of the battle casualty experience in Vietnam, but perhaps we did not go about it in the right way." Michael DeBakey tried to organize another effort in the late 1970s, but it too fell short.[133] Not until the 1990s did the MFUA successfully integrate a new cohort of veterans into its studies.

Denied a role in the medical activities of the Vietnam War, the MFUA expanded its activities in other ways. It approved new uses of the Twin Registry in 1971, including studies of risk factors in coronary heart disease, hereditary and environmental factors in dermatological conditions, and familial factors in early mortality. In addition, CEVFUS approved studies of amyotrophic lateral sclerosis and Hodgkin's disease. The committee also discussed how best to take advantage of the forthcoming automation of the VA Master Index, used for identifying veterans, linking VA and military files, and ascertaining mortality. The committee hoped to add this Master Index to the major MFUA rosters such as the twin and body-build registries. The new computer file, called BIRLS (for Beneficiary Identification and Records Locator Subsystem), ultimately became one of MFUA's main resources for the establishment and maintenance of research cohorts. Agency staff also secured funds during the year for preserving the Army diagnostic index to the Korean War on magnetic tape in order to ensure its availability for future use. Finally, the committee began a lengthy review of the Army's proposed modernization of the routine physical examination (MORPE) given to all new recruits, with hopes that the new examination would provide standardized baseline information for research in the history of disease and would be more easily retrievable by researchers.[134]

The early 1970s brought strained relations with the Veterans Administration. Beebe and Dunham met in early 1971 with Dr. Lyndon Lee, assistant chief medical director for research and education in medicine at the VA, to discuss an old problem. Lee, who had been the agency's scientific liaison officer with the VA for many years before being promoted to his new position, had urged the MFUA to expand its program of studies to the Vietnam generation. Praising the overall MFUA program, he nonetheless lamented the agency's low profile, particularly among armed forces staff. As the VA's assistant chief medical director, Lee "expressed a desire to have some interlocking of the Committee with the main VA advisory structure," on the theory that this organizational change would give the recommendations of CEVFUS more weight with the VA. He also suggested recommendations "better grounded in the realities of the VA situation," a proposal that could be implemented if his suggestions to have "men presently close to the VA" added to the committee were implemented.[135]

Reflecting on the meeting with Dr. Lee, Beebe wrote to his superior Dr. Charles Dunham, still new enough as Keith Cannan's replacement that he had not yet become familiar with the place of the Medical Follow-up Agency within the NRC structure. Beebe reminded Dunham of the history of the earlier Committee on Veterans Medical Problems, phased out by Dunham's predecessor when its "broader" mandate proved impossible for its role as advisory body for the MFUA. Lee, he clearly implied, wanted to return to the earlier VA–NRC relationship, but Beebe cautioned against changing "the mission of the present Committee without a pretty good discussion of the reasons therefor," and without verification that it would be in the best interests of the Medical Follow-up Agency's program as well as those of the VA. If nothing else, Lee's requirements required adding several more clinical investigators to the committee, either at the expense of the existing disciplines represented there or at the cost of having to expand the committee.[136]

The CEVFUS meeting to discuss these matters lasted more than six hours, one of the longest on record. At this meeting, it appeared that Dunham's ideas meshed with Lee's plans for the committee. Dunham wanted a committee that approximated the active policy-setting oversight functions common to the NRC organization. If Lee and Dunham expected the committee to remake itself so quickly, however, they had grossly miscalculated. CEVFUS members expressed their unwillingness to take an "aggressive" stand in the development of the program, preferring instead to "encourage the kinds of studies that seem best suited to the opportunity presented by the military-veteran experience." So far removed was the committee from day-to-day operational thinking that its members declined to consider funding prospects for future proposals, on the somewhat dubious grounds that "worthwhile proposals would always find support." The committee effectively ceded to MFUA staff the basic program-setting responsibility that Dunham clearly had hoped the CEVFUS would seize. For his part, Lee's plan to return to the old MFUA–VA relationship was also denied. The committee expressed a desire to "recommend policy" to the VA, but only as that policy affected Medical Follow-up Agency matters.[137]

4

Recent Decades

With the loss of core support, the Medical Follow-up Agency (MFUA) relied on the Committee on Epidemiology and Veterans Follow-up Studies (CEVFUS) and on agencies such as the Veterans Administration (VA) to continue to generate worthwhile projects. In this context, a VA decision late in 1971 to review the operations of the MFUA appeared troublesome. The review, in fact, turned out well: reviewers were favorably impressed with MFUA's general procedures and its record of useful studies. They urged the VA to raise its level of support for the agency, but criticized the committee for taking little initiative in suggesting studies.[138]

Gilbert Beebe himself was of two minds on this matter. On the one hand, he was at times attracted to a CEVFUS that would take a greater role in shaping the agency's program. On the other hand, he found the vagueness of the VA recommendations puzzling, feeling that they reflected Lyndon Lee's earlier attempts to reshape the committee to a model of his own design. Moreover, expanding the CEVFUS initiative would place even more demands on a staff that was already overburdened. The Executive Committee of the National Research Council's (NRC's) Division of Medical Sciences Executive Committee echoed Beebe's sentiments, urging him to go slow, not to risk the flexibility that the MFUA's current organization gave it. However, the question of sources for MFUA studies was by no means closed. A study in 1977 found that only 2 of the 57 "R projects" (active studies, not mere planning studies) funded at the time were committee inspired, 34 came from government agencies, 13 from university investigators, and 7 from MFUA staff.[139]

Other outside agencies offered proposals that had the potential to change the MFUA's mission dramatically. The National Institutes of Health's (NIH's) National Heart and Lung Institute (NHLI, later the National Heart, Lung and Blood Institute [NHLBI]) wrote to Beebe and the MFUA in early 1972, mentioning NHLI's interest in "maximizing the return" on its field studies by "providing the means for follow-up studies of prognosis and outcome through a central registry and follow-up mechanism." Beebe recalled a similar suggestion made some years earlier by Michael DeBakey in relation to the ongoing collaborative clinical trials sponsored by NIH. At the time, the MFUA felt ill-equipped to handle the problems of the "uncharted sea" that would arise in this new function and did not act on the suggestion.[140]

This time, the offer came from the NHLI itself, with implicit promise of funding, thus giving the MFUA an opportunity to broaden its program beyond the study of the mortality and morbidity of veterans. Although CEVFUS and MFUA staff gave serious consideration to the offer, they ultimately rejected it. As Beebe wrote to the NHLI's associate director, agency interest was piqued in part by the thought that this offer would allow the MFUA to refocus its efforts on morbidity studies, since follow-up data on veterans who were not using the VA system were increasingly limited in the decades since World War II. Only hospital insurance plans seemed likely prospects to offer these kinds of data in the near future, and there would be confidentiality problems in acquiring such information. This would not be an issue with the NHLI proposal. The committee's conclusion, however, was that the "technical means to facilitate studies of morbidity on a national basis did not now exist nor were they in near prospect. The task of attempting to develop methods applicable nationally would be very large, and is probably beyond the strength of the Follow-up Agency." Beebe did note some interest within CEVFUS in morbidity studies on a smaller scale and some flexibility on the question of extending the MFUA program beyond the veteran population in cases "where the value and feasibility of studies on other groups were assured." NHLI, however, chose to consider the book closed on MFUA involvement in this effort on any scale.[141] Despite this decision, NHLI played a key role in funding the assembly and maintenance of the NAS–NRC Twin Registry for many years.

Although MFUA spurned NHLI's proposal, the agency and the committee did gain some important additions in 1972. First, the agency found a replacement for Dean Nefzger: Dennis Robinette, a biological statistician who remained on staff until his death in 1992 and played an important role in program continuity during his tenure with the MFUA (see Box 10). The following year, Dr. James E. Norman, a statistician formerly at the University of Georgia, joined the MFUA staff. At its 1972 meeting, the committee also decided to appoint two subcommittees. One was an ad hoc subcommittee on the Army's ongoing modernization of the routine physical examination (MORPE) efforts. Of more importance was the appointment of a Subcommittee on Surgical Problems, charged to "review the

---

BOX 10
Study of Splenectomy and Subsequent Mortality

"A long-term follow-up of 740 American servicemen splenectomised because of trauma during the 1939–1945 war showed significant excess mortality from pneumonia and ischemic heart disease. Mortality from cirrhosis was also increased, but not significantly. The findings confirm that the risk of fatal infections is increased by asplenia; however, the risk of cancer was not increased, as it is in some other immunodeficiency states. Post-splenectomy thrombocytosis and hypercoagulability may account for the increased risk of fatal myocardial ischaemia in this group" (see Robinette and Fraumeni, 1977).

These findings provided the principal basis for establishing Department of Defense policy regarding the nondeployable status of splenectomized individuals to tropical areas of the world. The findings of thrombocytosis, hypercoagulability, and increased risk of mortality due to ischemic heart disease preceded by a decade the studies on the value of aspirin in preventing myocardial infarction.

Selected Reference
Robinette, C.D., Fraumeni, J.F. Splenectomy and subsequent mortality in veterans of the 1939–45 war. *Lancet* 2(July):127–129, 1977.

---

scientific and clinical needs for information obtainable only by means of follow-up studies based on the surgical experience in Vietnam." Dunham appointed Dr. Stuart Roberts, who had been the Army's surgical consultant in Vietnam, to head the subcommittee, with membership including Michael DeBakey and others.[142]

At the annual meeting of the division of medical sciences in April 1972, members of the Executive Committee found, somewhat to their surprise, that this low-profile organization within the division was a "very active group." Indeed, during 1972, the Medical Follow-up Agency activities continued at a high rate. CEVFUS approved two new twin studies that year. One was a pilot study of a new effort in the ongoing examination of smoking and twins; the other was a study of headache patterns in twin pairs in relation to zygosity. A non-twins study that was approved was part of the continuing work on amyotrophic lateral sclerosis, a follow-up effort to chart its course and that of other motor neuron diseases over time and to search for prognostic indicators. Other ongoing studies included one on body build and mortality, using a study of 105,000 men being discharged from military service in 1946 developed by a group of physical anthropologists. MFUA investigators retrieved the data from the study and performed a mortality analysis of the more than 7,000 confirmed deaths in the cohort.[143]

The agency continued these commitments in a period of organizational uncertainty. In 1972, the NRC was undergoing one of a periodic series of reorganization efforts as it attempted to mold its mission to suit changing national needs. In a ripple effect from this larger effort, the NRC ordered that all committees institute more regular rotation, including CEVFUS. Division of Medical Sciences Chairman Charles Dunham therefore brought in new committee leadership, appointing Dr. Richard Remington, a biostatistician and associate dean for research at the University of Texas School of Public Health, to the chairmanship. Remington was chosen in part because he had previously served as chairman of one of the VA research committees and thus was acceptable to Dr. Lee of the VA. Dr. Brian MacMahon's relationship with the Medical Follow-up Agency did not end, however; he returned to the chairmanship of the committee in later years.[144]

At Dr. Remington's first meeting as CEVFUS chairman in January 1973, he proposed changes in committee procedures. He called for more use of outside opinions of the scientific merit of technical proposals, more committee discussion of policy, a more active committee role in seeking MFUA funding, and more frequent meetings.

For the first time since CEVFUS had been formed, the committee heard investigators, instead of MFUA staff, present their own proposals. Dr. Charlotte Silverman of the Public Health Service became the first female outside investigator to propose a study to the agency when she presented a proposal on exposure to microwave radiation (see Box 11). Like the other proposals presented that day by the investigators themselves, the project was approved, although this procedural innovation was rarely repeated thereafter. The other two proposals were a study of long-term effects of arsenic as used in the treatment of syphilis in World War II and a 30-year clinical follow-up of selected demyelinating diseases, related to the ongoing multiple sclerosis effort. The two major planning studies discussed that day both involved investigators who, although able to manage all other aspects of a study with their own resources, needed help in using the veterans' record files at the St. Louis center. Although the Medical Follow-up Agency had gone along with similar studies where appropriate to the workload of the St. Louis staff, it expressed reservations about these two studies. In particular, the study entitled "Prospective Studies of Mortality from Cerebrovascular Disease in Selected Groups of Pre-World War II and World War II Veterans," proposed by former MFUA staffer Dean Nefzger, required that no fewer than 120,000 records be examined over a period of three to four years. After lengthy discussions, the MFUA staff concluded that there was no way the agency could commit so much staff time to this effort without a fundamental reordering of its priorities. The committee therefore declined Nefzger's proposal and accepted the other, much smaller one.[145]

THE FIRE IN SAINT LOUIS

Progress on MFUA projects was severely impeded when, on July 12, 1973, a fire broke out at the Military Personnel Records Center in St. Louis. There were no injuries, but the fire, which burned sporadically for the next three days, hampered all MFUA studies requiring World War II-era medical details from Army hospital

---

BOX 11
Health Effects of Occupational Exposure to
Microwave Radiation (RADAR)

Concerns about the cancer-causing effects of nonionizing electromagnetic radiation increased in the aftermath of newspaper stories linking cellular phone use to cancer risk. Because cellular telephones are a relatively recent invention, however, a long-term follow-up of cell phone users is obviously not yet possible. Nevertheless, it has been possible to study the long-term health effects following exposure to microwave radiation, nonionizing radiation that occupies a similar place in the electromagnetic spectrum. Thus the Medical Follow-up Agency was asked to bring up to date an earlier study on the long-term effects of exposure to microwave radiation.

In 1980, the MFUA published the results of a mortality follow-up of 40,000 Navy servicemen, of whom half had maximum opportunity for exposure to microwave radiation and the other half had minimum opportunity. The study compared the health experiences of those who repaired radar equipment (maximum opportunity) with those who operated it (minimum opportunity); all subjects were graduates of Navy technical schools in 1950 to 1954. Although a direct measure of physical exposure could not be determined, relative exposure was scaled using occupation, length of time in occupation, and power of the RADAR units aboard the ship on which a subject served.

The study found no adverse health effects as reflected in mortality, military hospitalization or VA hospitalization, or VA disability compensation rates. The study's results were published not long after those from a study of persons who were exposed to microwave radiation while serving in the U.S. Embassy in Moscow, which found no appreciable health differences in those exposed to what were thought to be low levels of microwave radiation. A further mortality follow-up, which is to gather an additional 20 years of data, is under way as the MFUA enters its sixth decade.

Selected Reference

Robinette, C.D., Silverman, C., Jablon, S. Effects upon health of occupational exposure to microwave radiation (RADAR). *American Journal of Epidemiology* 112:39–53 1980.

---

charts or epidemiologic data from Army personnel records. The MFUA staff in St. Louis was forced to relocate during the laborious process of cleaning and restoring the building. In May 1974, Seymour Jablon surveyed the situation for the committee: 80 percent of the Army personnel and medical records from World War II and the Korean War were lost. Mortality follow-up studies were still possible with the continued existence of the Beneficiary Identification and Records Locator Subsystem (BIRLS) on magnetic tape. Studies that aimed at epidemiologic factors or required review of clinical records were largely no longer feasible.

The fire forced the MFUA to rely more heavily on Navy records and less on the Army records with which it was so comfortable. "[O]ne of the great values of the program was precisely that it had been possible to study reasonably large groups of men with relatively rare conditions, and this would no longer be possible," the committee noted. Indeed, except for studies where the indexing was already complete, it became very difficult to develop studies for some diseases.[146]

As part of his effort to hold more meetings, Remington convened the committee for a second time in 1973. The committee faced a changed external environment with the completion of the NRC reorganization. The Medical Follow-up Agency and CEVFUS now formed parts of the new Assembly of Life Sciences. The old Division of Medical Sciences continued to exist but as a much reduced entity. With the retirement of Charles Dunham, the MFUA staff and CEVFUS had to get to know an all-new hierarchy, including Leonard Laster, executive director of the new Assembly of Life Sciences.

In addition to discussing the new organizational structure, the committee devoted the bulk of its time at the second 1973 meeting to its subcommittee on MORPE and the revision of the Army's induction examination. The subcommittee focused on the data for cardiovascular research that could be retrieved from the revised examination. The larger committee chose to accept the subcommittee's report without forwarding it to the Army staff on the grounds that the proposal was not "original" enough.[147]

In 1975, the issue of the MORPE program arose again. Since the Army had delegated MORPE interests to the Air Force, the current effort to modernize the examination system was directed to Armed Forces Entrance Examination Station (AFEES) operation, with a pilot run to commence at the Baltimore AFEES in 1975. Although the committee expressed its regret that no greater effort was being made to standardize examination procedures, yielding universally applicable data, it was encouraged by the fact that the new record system might make it possible to maintain a data base on those who had been rejected. Such a data base would be useful in controlling for the so-called healthy veteran syndrome, which postulated that men on the MFUA's veteran rosters were less susceptible to disease than the general population since they had passed the physical examination on induction. MFUA staff officer Robert J. Keehn suggested that new data arising from MORPE and the AFEES modernization impelled the committee to take the lead in the establishment of data bases for future studies, rather than relying on data bases laid down and preserved by others.[148]

As it worked with the subcommittees, the MFUA could also report progress in a number of ongoing projects. The group at the VA responsible for research on alcoholism approached the MFUA, anxious to set up long-term studies of alcoholism in association with the armed forces but confused as to how to proceed. Changing attitudes within the military regarding alcoholism—that is, considering it a disease worthy of treatment rather than a reason for summary dismissal—opened up new possibilities for research.[149] Plans were being made to update prisoner of war (POW) mortality for the POW study through 1972, to verify if the excess mortality reported in the first follow-up of World War II Pacific prisoners and Korean War prisoners continued to level off as it had in the 1965 results. Twin studies centering on schizophrenia, cancer morbidity, headache, and economic success were under way. A final report on the epidemiology of herniated lumbar disks was in preparation, following presentation of a preliminary report on this work at the annual meeting of the Society for Epidemiologic Research in May 1972. Also, the ongoing study of multiple sclerosis cases diagnosed in World War II entered a new phase as investigators made efforts to trace the course and prognosis of the disease for 30 years after its diagnosis. Three new studies were approved in late 1973, including a longitudinal study of cardiovascular disease, an examination of childhood cancer in relation to prenatal irradiation, and a series of related epidemiologic studies of various conditions for evidence of later death from cancer among World War II veterans.[150]

In 1974, despite the damage done to the MFUA program by the St. Louis fire, the agency made important strides in other areas. The committee met the new executive director of the Assembly of Life Sciences, Dr. Leonard Laster, who expressed approval of the Medical Follow-up Agency's history and current procedures, and promised not to get in the agency's way. He did, however, affirm a commitment to increase committee turnover, meaning that new CEVFUS members had to learn the ropes very quickly. In later years, this problem was handled by rotating a fixed group of members.

The etiquette of statistical reporting also commanded the committee's attention in 1974. The committee heard discussions of problems with the VA's new BIRLS system. CEVFUS unofficially affirmed its support for the creation of the National Death Index being proposed by the National Center for Health Statistics, a more efficient way to determine mortality for large numbers of people than the then-current system of making inquiries of each state. The National Death Index came on-line in 1979 and eventually proved to be very helpful in the work of the Medical Follow-up Agency.[151]

Updating the core statistical resources of the agency remained a common theme in the mid-1970s. Jablon continued his efforts to adapt Navy records to MFUA uses, reporting to CEVFUS on his progress at their 1975 meeting. The Navy records were problematic in that no machine-readable diagnostic index to the Navy files for World War II existed, making these files extremely difficult to use. Although "F card files," containing information on admissions to Navy hospitals during World War II existed, they were filed sequentially by hospital and year of admission, and the cards were not punched. When Jablon took a sample of 1,500 cards and examined them for diagnosis, he found that the top two diagnoses were for infectious and parasitic diseases and for acute infections of the respiratory system. Hence, reliance on these records meant a shift in program emphasis to tropical diseases and other common naval ailments. After studying the matter for some time, Jablon estimated in 1976 that $100,000 would be needed for punching items and producing a magnetic tape file in diagnostic sequence for MFUA use, if the agency wished to organize and preserve all of the Navy cards. With support from the National Cancer Institute, 6 million Navy hospital admissions from 1944 to 1945 had been preserved on magnetic tape by the early 1980s.[152]

Although Dr. Zdenek Hrubec's absence during 1974, on a year's detachment at the Karolinska Institute in Stockholm, meant that no new twin studies were launched, the committee approved a new statement of "Principles Which Govern Use of the NAS–NRC Twin Registry." Among the innovative studies in the area was one by Dr. Paul Taubman. Taubman, an economist rather than an epidemiologist, used the roster of twins to generate data on genetics and earnings. Of 6,000 twin pairs, 2,500 pairs responded to a questionnaire. Taubman ultimately reported his results in a monograph as well as several journal articles.[153]

AT MID-DECADE

In 1975, CEVFUS discussed the future of the MFUA program. Dr. Robert W. Miller of the National Cancer Institute noted a retreat from the emphasis on studies of trauma. In fact, no studies of trauma were being undertaken, in part because methods of treating trauma in the 1970s were so different from those used in World War II.

As chairman of the MFUA's advisory committee, Richard Remington urged the agency to approach the Department of Defense for possible consultation efforts, to tailor its program to better fit the needs of the VA, and to try to publish an account of its program in a journal such as the *New England Journal of Medicine*. Few of these proposals were carried out, however.[154]

As a result, in the bicentennial year 1976, the MFUA faced a number of internal and external challenges. As Gilbert Beebe prepared to turn over the reins of the agency upon reaching the age of 65 in 1977, he surveyed the changes in the kind of epidemiologic studies that the MFUA undertook in the 1970s as opposed to the 1940s. He noted a number of complicating factors, including the 1973 fire, the difficulty in contacting the veterans due to the passage of time, the national concern with privacy and confidentiality, the fragmentation of VA files in numerous locations, the destruction of the previous automatic link between VA hospitalization and the claims folder, the growing resistance of veterans to questionnaires or other studies, and the numerous non-VA alternatives open to veterans seeking hospitalization. On the positive side, such developments as the creation of magnetic tape files, the development of epidemiologic knowledge, the creation of BIRLS, the adoption of the Social Security number as the military service serial number, the growing number of veterans, and increasing concern with the effects of environmental factors on human health aided the MFUA program.

One matter that occupied Beebe's attention was the passage of the 1974 Privacy Act by Congress.[155] Beebe prevailed on National Academy of Sciences (NAS) President Philip Handler to bring the committee's concerns to the attention of the Privacy Protection Study Commission in connection with the commission's consideration of regulations to enforce the Privacy Act. Committee members feared that these regulations would make epidemiological studies of the sort that the Medical Follow-up Agency had conducted in the past impossible; confidentiality concerns would preclude the release of patient data by the relevant agencies. Handler wrote the commission's executive director that he hoped its "deliberations on the uses of records will give adequate representation to scientific uses of records in furthering public health." With Handler's support, the MFUA successfully persuaded the commission to issue regulations that made allowance for the use of medical records for the agency's kinds of epidemiological studies.[156]

THE ASSEMBLY OF LIFE SCIENCES

Closer to home, however, things did not go so well. The Executive Committee of the recently created Assembly of Life Sciences (ALS) experienced as much trouble getting used to the MFUA as had some of its predecessors in the Division of Medical Sciences. In examining the MFUA program in 1976, the Executive Committee called particular attention to the ongoing surgical adjuvant cancer therapy trials, probably the most atypical part of the agency's program. Some Executive Committee members thought the work "too pedestrian and unproductive to justify continuation." Recognizing that it was an ongoing effort, the Executive Committee approved it for fiscal year 1977 with the stipulation that CEVFUS should review the question of continuing MFUA involvement in the series of trials. At its May 25, 1976, meeting, CEVFUS agreed to appoint an ad hoc subcommittee, headed by Dr. Thomas C. Chalmers of the Mount Sinai School of Medicine, to review the matter. Chalmers's subcommittee recommended that the MFUA continue its collaborative role in the studies. He based his recommendations on the finding that although the trials had produced largely negative results thus far point, hope for more successful therapies still existed. Moreover, the protocols were well constructed and the studies well executed, statistical aspects of the design and analysis were of high quality, the work was efficiently managed with little use of precious staff time, and working relations with the coinvestigators were excellent. Calling the trials "an appropriate form of diversification for the MFUA," and arguing that "the future of MFUA collaboration should not be contingent upon showing positive results," the committee voted to send the Chalmers subcommittee report to the ALS Executive Committee as its reply to the concern about cancer trials.[157]

The matter did not end there. Paul Marks, Columbia's vice president for health sciences and former chairman of the Division of Medical Sciences, became a critic of the Medical Follow-up Agency within the ALS Executive Committee. In response, Beebe, Jablon, and Remington proposed that Marks and other representatives of the Executive Committee organize a "visiting committee" that would make an informal site visit to examine the MFUA program and its relation to the larger ALS unit. Alvin Lazen, associate executive director of the ALS went so far as to propose formally the creation and mandate of such a committee to Dr. Marks, who would head it. However, Marks did not convene the committee. When the ALS Executive Committee considered the MFUA's contract proposals in 1977, "things went badly," particularly the discussion of blood pressure and multiple sclerosis projects. Beebe worried that he was leaving the agency at a time when the program was vulnerable to attack from within the NRC. Finally, a review committee was appointed by ALS Chairman James Ebert, a biologist with the Carnegie Institution, to "recapitulate the history of MFUA, identify the nature of questions now being raised concerning the Agency and determine how the panel can best address the questions." The presence of both MacMahon and Remington on the six-man panel ensured that the agency would receive a favorable hearing, and Beebe could retire from the Medical Follow-up Agency knowing that, at least for the time being, it was not in danger from within.[158]

In 1976, Beebe's imminent retirement, as well as a sense that the agency's program was not growing rapidly enough, led Remington to assign to various committee members the task of assessing the future needs of specific disciplines for Medical Follow-up Agency studies. Dr. Robert H. Felix of the Bi-State Regional Medical Program in St. Louis and the distinguished former head of the National Institute of Mental Health was assigned to consider the field of psychiatry; Dr. DeBakey, surgery; and Dr. Reuel A. Stallones of the University of Texas School of Public Health, cardiovascular disease. At the December 1976 meeting, Dr. Stallones presented his report on cardiovascular disease and the MFUA program, recommending that a summary of the agency's usefulness as a resource be reprinted periodically in the *American Journal of Epidemiology* and that the agency seek special funding from the NHLBI for planning cardiovascular disease studies. DeBakey presented a number of potential surgical studies that could be undertaken by the agency, including follow-up of studies done in its earliest days, as well as some new ideas such as a study of men with spinal cord injuries. Since Felix was unable to complete his overview of the psychiatric field due to illness, Dr. Ransom J. Arthur of the Neuropsychiatric Institute at the University of California at Los Angeles (UCLA) took his place.[159]

SEYMOUR JABLON IN CHARGE

After Beebe retired in 1977, Seymour Jablon took over the day-to-day operations of the Medical Follow-up Agency, as well as those of the Atomic Bomb Casualty Commission's (ABCC's) successor agency, the Radiation Effects Research Foundation (RERF). Jablon had been with the agency almost since the beginning and was a well-respected statistician. As such he possessed the necessary experience to run the agency. Unfortunately, he presided over a difficult

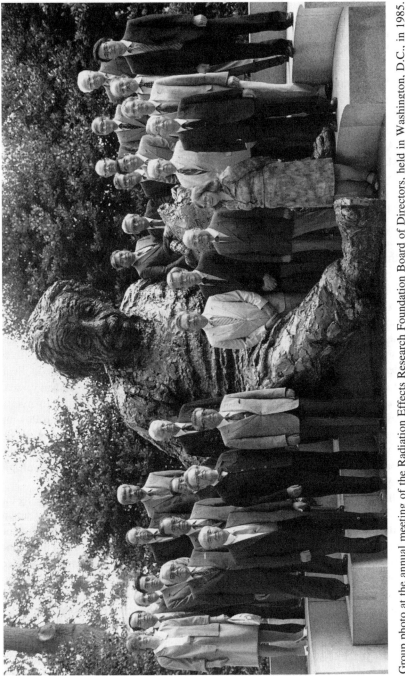

63

Group photo at the annual meeting of the Radiation Effects Research Foundation Board of Directors, held in Washington, D.C., in 1985. Photo courtesy of Dr. Gilbert Beebe.

period for the agency. The committee began to meet increasingly rarely and considered fewer new program initiatives. Funding became increasingly problematic as the 1980s began. The country's continued economic problems affected the Medical Follow-up Agency during this period, as it did most entities that relied on government funding. However, the agency could point to numerous completed manuscripts, and publication levels remained healthy; only in 1982 did agency projects yield as few as four published manuscripts. Other years in this troubled period saw almost three times as many articles printed in respected journals by agency staff or investigators.[160]

As Remington reached the end of his chairmanship in 1977, he looked over the Medical Follow-up Agency and noted some of the ongoing limitations of the agency's efforts. By now the litany of complaints was familiar. Extensive pilot work was often required to assess project feasibility and cost. The very breadth of the MFUA mission also left it no specific focus. The fragmentation, and even obsolescence, of source documents and the extensive use of non-VA hospitals by veterans lessened the usefulness of the veteran cohort over time. Moreover, its funding pattern left the agency unable to plan effectively, and the weakness of the agency's links to the larger scientific community meant that this funding pattern was unlikely to change soon.[161]

Yet, the agency continued to take on new projects. Studies exploring the relationships between immunological abnormalities of various kinds and subsequent cancer were undertaken in collaboration with the National Cancer Institute. Twin projects, including topics as diverse as genetic variations in fluoride effects on dental caries, cardiovascular disease, Parkinson's disease, and alcoholism, were approved in the last two meetings of the 1970s. A study of Navy radar workers, which found no measurable health effects from exposure to microwaves, and a study of World War II veterans with limb amputations following trauma (see Box 12) which found excessive mortality from cardiovascular disease, were completed. CEVFUS also approved pilot studies on alcoholism among veterans and the potential relationship between household pets and multiple sclerosis.[162]

In 1982, Dr. Lazen of the Academy of Life Sciences proposed reorganizing the MFUA as a more broad-based epidemiological organization, emphasizing "activities of a more traditional, advisory kind," such as the agency's review of the protocol for a study of health effects of phenoxy herbicides in Vietnam and its still-nascent entry into the area of atomic veterans. In part because of Zed Hrubec's departure in 1981, Jablon found himself understaffed as well as underfunded. Jablon realized that much of the work Lazen prescribed for this proposed committee on epidemiology was already being done by other groups in universities and government. "There may be occasional cases in which our own talents and expertise surpass those available to any other group," he wrote, "but I cannot think of any offhand." Lazen backed down. Jablon, after all, had history on his side.[163]

For want of core support with which to pay meeting costs, CEVFUS went

---

BOX 12
Study of Cardiovascular Disease Following
Traumatic Limb Amputations

Although the Medical Follow-up Agency is not involved directly in decisions affecting disability compensation following military service, occasionally the results of its studies will have an effect on compensation. A congressionally mandated follow-up of mortality after traumatic amputation, published in 1980, was just such a study. The study followed almost 4,000 men who had had proximal amputations (i.e., knee or above, elbow or above) and compared their mortality experience with that of two comparison groups, a group with distal amputations (loss of part of hand or part of foot) and a group with disfiguring injuries.

The group of proximal amputees had significantly higher mortality from all causes, especially ischemic heart disease. Partly in response to the findings of this study, the Veterans Administration changed its policy with regard to the compensation of veterans with traumatic amputations.

Selected Reference

Hrubec, Z., Ryder, R. Traumatic limb amputation and subsequent mortality from cardiovascular disease and other causes. *Journal of Chronic Disease* 33:239–250, 1980.

---

four years between meetings, from March 1979 until May 1983. In the meantime, the agency's staff completed studies on multiple sclerosis, Hodgkin's disease, and tetrachloroethane and cancer, and the pilot study on the relationship between household pets and multiple sclerosis. The National Cancer Institute decided, after 25 years, to terminate the cancer chemotherapy trials that had caused such enmity between the MFUA and the ALS. Studies in progress in 1983 included a morbidity update for World War II and Korean War POWs, a prospective study of testicular cancer, study of the possible long-term effects of short-term exposure to chemical agents in a series of tests at Edgewood Arsenal (see Box 13), an epidemiologic study of mesothelioma and employment, and a protocol prepared for the VA on the health effects of Agent Orange.[164]

When CEVFUS next met in 1983, the committee approved all but one of the projects before it. Accepted twin studies involved criminality, senile macular degeneration, and presenile dementia among the roster of twins. Also, the VA approached the MFUA with a proposal to develop a Vietnam-Era service twin register, which the VA ultimately took over but not before much work had been done by MFUA staff. Non-twins proposals that CEVFUS approved included a study of mortality patterns in veterans with psychiatric diagnoses in World War II, three studies of multiple sclerosis, and a follow-up of an earlier hepatitis study.[165]

From the late 1970s through most of the 1980s, the only part of the federal

---

BOX 13
Follow-up of Veterans Experimentally Exposed to
Chemical Agents

Interest in the effects of exposure to anticholinesterase agents—for example, the nerve gas sarin—grew in response to reports of the possible exposure of Persian Gulf War veterans to such agents. Thus, the Medical Follow-up Agency was asked to conduct an additional long-term follow-up study of a group of soldiers who had been experimentally exposed to chemical agents in the past.

The MFUA had already conducted an initial follow-up of some 6,720 Army soldiers who were enrolled in a program of experimental exposure to chemical warfare and other agents at the Edgewood Arsenal, Maryland, between 1955 and 1975. A three-volume report was issued in 1980; the last volume—of which MFUA staff had lead authorship—dealt with the current health status of test subjects, including 1,581 men exposed to anticholinesterase compounds such as GA (tabun), GB (sarin), GD (soman), GF, and VX. Subjects exposed to such compounds did not differ substantially from those exposed to other compounds or from unexposed comparison individuals in their replies to questions about current health. However, given the limitations of the study design, only large health effects were likely to be uncovered.

As this volume goes to print, the MFUA is waiting word on funding of the proposed study to continue follow-up of these same subjects. The new study, however, will be of a more focused nature than the earlier investigation; in particular, research is expected to focus on the neurological and neuropsychological sequelae of low-level exposures to organophosphate pesticides, which are somewhat similar in their chemical action to the nerve agents tested at Edgewood Arsenal.

Selected Reference

National Research Council. *Possible Long-Term Health Effects of Short-Term Exposure to Chemical Agents,* Volume 3: *Final Report: Current Health Status of Test Subjects.* Washington, D.C.: National Academy Press, 1985.

---

budget that showed steady growth was the Department of Defense (DOD). With MFUA funding constricted in all directions, Jablon looked to this department for new studies. The MFUA and the DOD were an ideal fit. The Defense Department sought experts to study the exposure of various veteran cohorts to atomic radiation. Jablon's experience with the ABCC and some related, smaller-scale studies in the 1970s, gave him and his staff experience needed to carry out such work. Beginning in 1978, the Medical Follow-up Agency and the Defense Department's Defense Nuclear Agency entered into a series of contracts that would last into the 1990s. These radiation contracts were almost the agency's predominant means of support for much of the early 1980s. They were not without political conflicts. Jablon's first study, on the incidence of cancer among veterans who entered Hiroshima and Nagasaki in 1945 immediately after atomic bombs leveled these two Japanese cities, found no unusual incidence of multiple myeloma among these "atomic veterans." However, the protocols and the conclusions of the study came under such intense scrutiny from Capitol Hill and the press, that Jablon agreed to do the study again.[166]

Other related studies undertaken by the agency concentrated on servicemen who were present at a number of atmospheric atomic bomb tests between 1946 and 1962, with code names such as SMOKY and CROSSROADS. A series of MFUA subcommittees organized the protocols for these epidemiologic studies, all of which reported results similar to the original Hiroshima and Nagasaki studies. Disappointed veterans groups criticized Jablon, who publicly defended the method behind the studies but privately admitted that they were not the best kind of science. Since the agency needed the money, Jablon continued to take the lead on these studies well after he left the agency staff. His position in the atomic test exposure studies continued until Kenneth Shine, president of the Institute of Medicine, removed him from the CROSSROADS study in 1993 under pressure from atomic veteran groups who were hoping for study results closer to their own, less scientific, predispositions.[167] The studies continued however to demonstrate the essential soundness of Jablon's methodologies and conclusions.

Even without substantial funds, the agency remained "actively involved" in building a new Vietnam-Era Twin Registry, as well as in the study of yellow fever vaccine and hepatitis in World War II veterans (see Box 14), and the ongoing POW work. In building the registry the agency ran into troubles with the Social Security Administration that were reminiscent of its problems with the Federal Bureau of Investigations two decades earlier. Social Security numbers had become standardized military case markers, replacing old serial numbers in the post-Korean War period. When the agency knew a veteran's name and date of birth, it needed the veteran's Social Security number. If it knew the veteran's name and Social Security number, it still required the date of birth. Both processes were easy enough to automate, but the Social Security Administration refused to cooperate on grounds of legal difficulties over the matter of disclosure. Failure to obtain these data made using the National Death Index and obtaining a mailing address from the Internal Revenue Service more difficult. In 1986, however, the Social Security Administration published a routine-use statement for the VA that allowed the Medical Follow-up Agency to gain more ready access to the data it needed.[168]

Between 1983 and 1985, the MFUA completed a study of mesothelioma and employment, intended to improve understanding of the health risks presented by exposure to asbestos and other fibers, the data for which were then being analyzed by the National Cancer Institute. Even as the agency expanded the Twin Registry to Vietnam veterans, it mailed new health questionnaires to the living members of the older registry (approximately 24,000 of the original 32,000 members remained in 1985) and planned future studies of diabetes and of possible links between handedness and neurological disease.

At this point in the agency's history, proposals tended to focus on diseases

BOX 14
A 41-Year Follow-up of
Hepatitis B Epidemic in the U.S. Army

Between late 1941 and early 1942 an epidemic of jaundice occurred in Army training camps across the United States. The epidemic was later determined to have resulted from the inoculation of an estimated 330,000 persons with contaminated yellow fever vaccine. The subsequent discovery of hepatitis B (HBV) provided an opportunity to (1) verify that the infectious agent was HBV and (2) test the hypothesis that adult infection with the virus in the United States leads to a carrier state with a high risk of hepatocellular carcinoma (HCC). Three groups totaling nearly 70,000 men were the subjects of a cohort study: group 1 was comprised of men hospitalized with hepatitis in 1942; group 2 consisted of men who were subclinically infected in 1942 by virtue of their having received vaccine from a contaminated lot without developing clinical disease; and group 3 contained comparison individuals who entered service after use of the contaminated vaccine had been discontinued.

Approximately 200 men from each of these groups were located in 1985–1986 and their blood was tested for HBV markers. This serological survey demonstrated that the epidemic was caused by HBV infection: antibodies to HBV were detected in 98, 77, and 13 percent of groups 1, 2, and 3 respectively, while antibodies to hepatitis A were identified in similar percentages of each group. Only one carrier of the hepatitis B surface antigen marker, from group 1, was found in the 392 men from groups 1 and 2. The corresponding carrier rate of 0.3 percent contrasted markedly with the assumed rate of 5–10 percent following acute HBV infection.

The mortality follow-up study of the three cohorts covering the period 1946–1983, which employed expert review of clinical and pathology records to select HCC from among all causes of death so diagnosed, found only a slight excess in mortality due to HCC in group 2, but not in group 1, compared with group 3 comparison individuals. Mortality from nonalcoholic chronic liver disease was *lower* in group 2 than in group 3. A case-control study of 24 HCC cases and 63 control subjects drawn from Department of Veterans Affairs hospital discharge files yielded an estimated relative risk for HCC due to receipt of contaminated vaccine of 3.3 ($p = 0.06$). The slightly elevated risk estimates from the mortality study, and the suggestive excess in the small case-control study, are consistent with the established etiological role of HBV infection in liver cancer. The serology study provided a rationale for these results, demonstrating that in comparison to neonates, young children, and immunosuppressed individuals of any age, healthy adults seldom become carriers of acute HBV infection. The mortality study provided evidence that the risk of HCC following HBV infection is probably small.

Selected References

Norman, J.E., Beebe, G.W., Hoofnagle, J.H., Seeff, L.B. Mortality follow-up of the 1942 epidemic of hepatitis B in the U.S. Army. *Hepatology* 18:790–797, 1993.
Seeff, L.B., Beebe, G.W., Hoofnagle, J.H., Norman, J.E., et al. A serologic follow-up of the 1942 epidemic of post-vaccination hepatitis in the U.S. Army. *New England Journal of Medicine* 316:965–970, 1987.

and conditions of the elderly, a natural result of the advancing age of the World War II cohort at the heart of the MFUA program. Proposals during this time included studies of Alzheimer's disease and head injury, brain cancer in elderly men, radio-frequency radiation and cancer, and Vietnam veterans with spinal cord injury.[169]

In 1986, the MFUA emerged from the doldrums that had predominated during the early 1980s. During this time, two important staffing changes took place. Robert Keehn retired from the agency and Dr. William Page, a biostatistician on temporary assignment from the VA, joined the staff. Dr. Page eventually made the temporary assignment a permanent one and subsequently came to play an important role in the modern history of the agency. The National Cancer Institute proposed that the MFUA collaborate on studies of cancer epidemiology based on hospital clinical records. Dr. Richard Miller, the future director of the agency but then the director of Walter Reed Army Institute of Research's residency program in general preventive medicine, began work with the agency on AIDS studies, developing a follow-up study of HIV-positive military personnel.[170]

In 1987, the ALS commissioned yet another task force to review the work and mission of the MFUA. Chaired by Brian MacMahon, it produced a laudatory report, calling the MFUA a "national resource which should be maintained and strengthened." It recommended keeping the agency within the NRC, securing core funding from the NIH, the VA, and other key governmental agencies, and suggested an immediate search for a new director with the retirement of Seymour Jablon in October 1987. The task force also mentioned the need for greater ties to investigators in academia and government agencies, as well as the possibility of changing the agency's name to reflect the breadth of its mission.[171]

WILLIAM PAGE'S INTERIM

With Jablon leaving, Alvin Lazen, executive director of the Commission on Life Sciences (the new functional equivalent of the former ALS), appointed William Page as acting director of the MFUA, effective June 15, 1987. In addition to running the day-to-day affairs of the agency, Page continued to manage important components of the program. At first, it appeared that Page would indeed be a transition figure; CEVFUS membership was extended for a year in the fall of 1987 with the idea that "by that time more should be known about the future direction of the Medical Follow-up Agency." Circumstances contrived to make Page's "transition" acting directorship about half as long as Jablon's actual tenure, however.[172]

Despite the confusion associated with the leadership transition, the MFUA was clearly on its way back. Lack of core funding was a key dilemma, and Gilbert Beebe acted from his "advisory" role to provide it. In August 1987, he initiated discussions with staff of the Senate Veterans Affairs Committee concerning the status of the agency. Beebe acted because, even with more grant money coming to the agency in 1987, the staff in St. Louis was reduced to very small numbers and put on temporary leave. Beebe's Senate meeting produced a "workshop" review of the Medical Follow-up Agency by the Office of Technology Assessment (OTA), held at the request of the Senate Veterans Affairs Committee in 1988. In the meantime, Page reapplied for core funding from the agency's major grant sources. The MFUA made it past the worst of a particularly difficult time when the POW and cancer studies were renewed and new studies of atomic veterans and oil adjuvant vaccines were launched.[173]

In 1987, the Medical Follow-up Agency once again reported on numerous accomplishments. Three papers had been generated by the POW study. Work continued on projects related to the long-term effects of the 1942 hepatitis epidemic in the Army. The agency sought to determine the prevalence in victims of various hepatitis markers and to estimate their mortality rates, especially from liver cancer and other liver diseases. Various multiple sclerosis and twin projects were under way or planned, and planning was also being undertaken on a 33-year follow-up of Army recruits immunized with adjuvant influenza vaccine to determine if long-term problems could be associated with this vaccine. In the same year, the committee approved two new studies, one on nephrectomies performed subsequent to trauma and another on posttraumatic stress in riflemen.[174]

In the midst of this activity, the appearance of OTA's report in November 1988 became a crucial milestone in the Medical Follow-up Agency's recent history. OTA staff argued that the MFUA was too important to wither away and that only the presence of core funding from NIH, the VA, and the Department of Defense could keep this from happening. As a short-term solution, OTA recommended shared core support for the agency among these three governmental bodies, beginning with fiscal year 1990. OTA staff advocated immediate core funding of $100,000 to allow the agency to carry on its work and search for a strong director. Thereafter, it recommended a total of $500,000 per year over five years. OTA also suggested that the NAS amend its rules on competitive bidding to allow the MFUA to bid for contracts within its natural purview.[175]

In the same year, the MFUA again gained a new parent entity within the National Academy of Sciences. This time, however, it left the NRC entirely. The so-called Rosenblith committee, led by Walter Rosenblith of the Massachusetts Institute of Technology, decided to transfer the MFUA, along with the better-known Food and Nutrition Board, to the Institute of Medicine (IOM). The IOM, an entity analogous in the Academy structure to the National Academy of Engineering (NAE), had developed out of discussions in the 1960s regarding the need for a "National Academy of Medicine," led by Dr. Irvine Page of the Cleveland Clinic (no relation to William Page of the MFUA). The entity that became the IOM started as the Board on Medicine. After the 1972 NRC reorganization, the IOM became a full-fledged "sister" organization to the NAS, NRC, and NAE.

This medical branch of the National Academy of Sciences was by no means an illogical place for the MFUA's epidemiological methods, and Page found himself as comfortable there as he had been in the NRC.[176]

However, the IOM was as uncomfortable with the MFUA as the agency's other parental entities had been in its more than 40 years of existence. A site visit by two outside investigators to familiarize the IOM with the workings of the MFUA took place in 1989. Pronouncing themselves "shocked" to learn that the Medical Follow-up Agency's very existence was in peril (although they admitted to being previously unaware of its existence themselves), the investigators called for "important changes" so that the agency might "continue, or even perhaps become again, the national resource it was intended to be." To quell the "interim" feelings that they detected on the part of the staff (only about ten persons at that time), the investigators recommended that the MFUA fill the position of a permanent director as soon as possible, preferably with a physician or epidemiologist. They urged securing long-term core funding, subsequent staff growth, and computer upgrades and spoke of the need for the agency to reach out better to the scientific community and the VA.[177]

By 1990, the Medical Follow-up Agency was again pursuing an active mandate. The agency sponsored a conference on epidemiology in military and veteran populations, as a sort of sequel to the workshop held in 1988, even publishing the proceedings with Dr. Page as editor. Seventy people attended the conference, which was intended both to report on the work of the agency and to draw new investigators into its orbit. After two years of wrangling and arm twisting by Senator Alan Cranston (D-California) and other members of the Senate Committee on Veterans Affairs, some of it public, first the NIH and then the VA agreed to fund the core program of the MFUA. Page and his staff believed that the funding derived from these agencies was more than sufficient for planning activities as the MFUA continued to grow in size for the second time in its history.[178]

In 1990, CEVFUS met again to discuss the agency's program and discovered an abundant amount of research done under MFUA auspices. Staff reported on the completed POW questionnaire, which found depressive symptomatology in POWs at a level three to five times higher than expected in a comparable general population. A study of hepatitis B and liver cancer in World War II veterans discovered little incidence of liver cancer in the study group. Ongoing efforts featured an examination study of former POWs, two other hepatitis studies, the mineral oil adjuvant study, and a pilot study of World War II veteran death reporting. Studies that awaited funding included the HIV study, an examination of Korean hemorrhagic fever (see Box 15), a study of multiple sclerosis, three twin studies, and a follow-up of nuclear veterans. In addition, the committee heard discussions of the body build registry, posttraumatic stress disorder in World War II riflemen, Alzheimer's disease, and head injury.[179]

BOX 15
Study of Hemorrhagic Fever with
Renal Syndrome

Interest in hantavirus infection was abruptly stimulated by a 1993 outbreak of hantavirus pulmonary syndrome in the Four Corners area of the United States—with case fatality rates as high as 50 percent. A newly discovered hantavirus, ultimately named Sin Nombre, was determined to be the cause of the outbreak. This marked the first occurrence of severe, acute disease in the United States causally linked to a hantavirus. The Four Corners outbreak brought with it concerns about the presence of newly identified infectious disease agents in the United States, as well as concerns regarding the possible long-term sequelae of a disease of this severity.

During the Korean War (1951–1953), American troops were exposed to another hantavirus: Hantaan. The Hantaan virus disease, initially called Korean hemorrhagic fever (KHF), is probably contracted through inhalation of the infected urine, saliva, or feces of the striped field mouse, *Apodemus agrarius*. Although the disease has been known for decades, no data are available on its long-term sequelae among American survivors.

A study published in 1960, in which the medical records of 1,416 KHF cases and 831 comparison individuals (all white) were reviewed, found a small but significant increase in renal injury and genitourinary disease three to five years after the acute phase of KHF. The Medical Follow-up Agency is currently involved in a follow-up study to determine longer-term outcomes in the original cohort, including the frequency of end-stage renal disease.

The MFUA, in collaboration with the University of Minnesota School of Public Health and the Centers for Disease Control and Prevention, is conducting a study of the long-term health effects of KHF in military personnel. The purpose of this study is to compare morbidity and mortality data from 1,416 white and 187 nonwhite surviving KHF cases with 831 white and 99 nonwhite comparison individuals. The study is scheduled for completion in the year 2000.

Selected Reference

Rubini, M.E., Jablon, S., McDowell, M.E. Renal residuals of acute epidemic hemorrhagic fever. *Archives of Internal Medicine* 106(Sept.):378–387, 1960.

THE 1990s

The 1990s proved to be a decade of positive developments for the MFUA. In 1991, Page could report that core funding had been secured from the National Institutes of Health, the Department of Defense, and the Veterans Administration. Two years later, this was again jeopardized by indifference within the funding agencies, but a follow-up OTA study in 1994 persuaded all three agencies to provide the money. In 1991, the agency completed its study of Army recruits immunized with oil adjuvant influenza vaccine, finding no statistically significant adverse effects of the oil adjuvant. With core funding in hand, Page urged the committee to broaden the agency's horizons. He discussed pilot studies of Health Care Finance Administration hospitalization and Social Security Administration mortality records, as well as MFUA's various computer needs in both hardware and software. Among the new projects proposed in that year were a follow-up study of 1950 Air Force recruits infected with hepatitis C, a follow-up of the West Point Class of 1956, and studies using the Navy hospitalization files that Seymour Jablon had preserved on computer tape with funding from the National Cancer Institute more than a decade before.[180]

BOX 16
Health Consequences of Persian Gulf War Service

In the years following Operations Desert Shield and Desert Storm in 1990–1991, reports of illnesses among Gulf War veterans raised public concerns about a "mystery illness" in this population. In 1993, Congress mandated that the Department of Veterans Affairs (VA) and the Department of Defense (DOD) arrange with the Medical Follow-up Agency to review existing scientific, medical, and other information on the health consequences of military service in the Persian Gulf War. A committee was constituted to assess the activities of the VA and DOD and to make recommendations concerning the collection and maintenance of information useful for evaluating the health consequences of service in the Persian Gulf. The committee was also to weigh the scientific basis for an epidemiologic study or studies to evaluate the health consequences of this service.

The committee worked for two years, providing an interim report in January 1995, and a final report in late 1996. The interim report noted limitations in the usefulness of the VA Persian Gulf Health Registry, urged better coordination of research related to Gulf War illnesses, and suggested improvements in the design of future projects to include population-based studies. The recommendation of the final report emphasized the need for medical information systems in the VA and DOD that would permit a single, continuous, retrievable medical record for each service person, a goal echoed by the President of the United States in November 1997. The report noted the need to monitor environmental exposures during deployment to allow for rapid response and appropriate data collection. It also stressed the need for data to better identify risk factors for stress-related disorders and other health outcomes among military personnel.

Selected References

Institute of Medicine. Committee to Review the Health Consequences of Service During the Persian Gulf War. *Health Consequences of Service During the Persian Gulf War: Initial Findings and Recommendations for Immediate Action.* Washington, D.C.: National Academy Press, 1995.

Institute of Medicine. Committee to Review the Health Consequences of Service During the Persian Gulf War. *Health Consequences of Service During the Persian Gulf War: Recommendations for Research and Information Systems.* Washington, D.C.: National Academy Press, 1996.

William Page's tenure as acting director reached an end in 1992 with the appointment of Chris Howson as interim director. After the ensuing search, IOM leadership recruited Dr. Richard Miller from the Walter Reed Medical Center as the new director of the program in 1993. Coming from both a medical and a military background, Miller fit many of the stipulations for a successful director set forth by the site visit group shortly after Jablon left the agency. Miller continued efforts begun under both Page and Howson. One especially notable study begun under Howson was designed to monitor the health status of Persian Gulf veterans (see Box 16). The mere fact of this study indicated that the agency fit better into the 1990s than at any time in decades. Page, Howson, and Miller would not let the opportunity presented by the Gulf War slip the way the Vietnam War had through the fingers of the MFUA staff in the early 1970s.

Miller took steps to make the agency more visible within the IOM structure, successfully arguing that the MFUA's oversight group should be a board instead

---

BOX 17
Studies of Participants in
Atmospheric Tests of Nuclear Weapons

In 1976 the case report of a paratrooper diagnosed with acute myelocytic leukemia reached the Centers for Disease Control and Prevention (CDC). The paratrooper attributed the leukemia's occurrence to his presence at the test detonation of the nuclear device "SMOKY." Subsequent preliminary investigations by the CDC and others raised concerns about increased mortality rates due to leukemia among all participants in atmospheric nuclear weapons tests. In 1979, the Medical Follow-up Agency was commissioned to investigate mortality among individuals present at these tests. This investigation culminated in a National Research Council (NRC) report *Mortality of Nuclear Weapons Test Participants*, published in 1985.

This report examined the records of soldiers participating in at least one of five select nuclear weapons test series between 1951 and 1957. Researchers did not identify any statistically significant increase in mortality attributed to radiation-related disease (e.g., leukemia or other malignancies) among the individuals studied, other than those leukemias previously noted among SMOKY participants. However, in 1992 the U.S. General Accounting Office distributed a report concluding that the data provided by the Defense Nuclear Agency (DNA), and used by the MFUA in the preparation of its 1985 report, contained misclassification errors that rendered the study flawed. The MFUA was asked to redo its earlier research. This study, scheduled for completion in 1999, uses a DNA-corrected and updated participant list, a comparison group of military personnel who did not participate in the atomic tests, and the addition of mortality data for 10 years since the earlier publication.

Meanwhile, in 1996, the NRC published another MFUA report examining mortality among participants in atmospheric tests of nuclear weapons. This study (Johnson et al. 1996) compared the mortality of Navy personnel participating in the CROSSROADS test series with the mortality of those in a comparison group. Although the study found a small but statistically significant increase in mortality

of a committee. Looking toward the future, Miller and his staff envisioned a Medical Follow-up Agency that would balance ongoing follow-up as in the multiple sclerosis or POW studies, cutting-edge research as in the various twin studies, and politically delicate studies such as those of Persian Gulf veterans or of atomic veterans (see Box 17).[181]

CONCLUSION

Since its founding in 1946, the Medical Follow-up Agency has successfully met many challenges. The agency continues to contribute to the research community because of the ingenuity and resolve of researchers such as Dr. Michael DeBakey. DeBakey and Gilbert Beebe sensed the opportunity to create a medical organization that would be a force for good in post-World War II America by channeling the experience of the war into useful medical knowledge. Beebe and

among the participants, its findings did not support the hypothesis that radiation exposure was the cause.

In part as an outgrowth of the MFUA's reputation in the field of atmospheric test participant research, the Army surgeon general asked the MFUA to assemble an expert committee to review a set of proposed NATO guidelines for the exposure of soldiers to radiation doses that are well short of those that cause acute effects but that may carry the risk of subsequent cancers. The committee's interim report addressed the technical aspects of the NATO documents. In its final report the committee discussed an ethical framework for considering when to put soldiers at risk and what obligations might then follow. Although this last activity does not directly benefit the test participants, it may contribute to the military's avoidance of unnecessary radiation exposures in the future and may help to improve the decision-making and operating procedures in place to protect personnel in cases where exposure is deemed warranted.

Selected References

Institute of Medicine. A Review of the Dosimetry Data Available in the Nuclear Test Personnel Review (NTPR) Program: An Interim Letter Report of the Committee to Study the Mortality of Military Personnel Present at Atmospheric Tests of Nuclear Weapons. Washington, D.C.: National Academy Press, 1995.

Institute of Medicine. *An Evaluation of Radiation Exposure Guidance for Military Operations, Interim Report.* J.C. Johnson and S. Thaul (eds.). Washington, D.C.: National Academy Press, 1997.

Institute of Medicine. *Potential Radiation Exposure in Military Operations: Protecting the Soldier Before, During, and After.* S. Thaul and H. O'Maonaigh (eds.). Washington, D.C.: National Academy Press, 1999.

Johnson, J.C., Thaul, S., Page, W.F., Crawford, H. *Mortality of Veteran Participants in the CROSSROADS Nuclear Test.* Washington, D.C.: National Academy Press, 1996.

National Research Council. *Mortality of Nuclear Weapons Test Participants.* Washington, D.C.: National Academy Press, 1985.

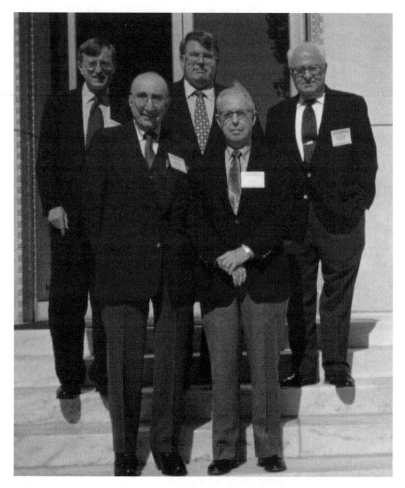

Past and present MFUA leadership gathered at the 50th Anniversary Meeting on October 16, 1996. From left to right, back row: Dr. William Page, Dr. Richard Miller, and Mr. Seymour Jablon; front row: Dr. Michael DeBakey and Dr. Gilbert Beebe. Photo courtesy of Dr. William Page.

his successors—Jablon, Page, Miller, and numerous others have fostered an entity flexible enough to mold itself to the times but resolute enough to overcome the numerous obstacles in its path. Although DeBakey and Beebe thought the agency would help guide clinical practice, the entity they created instead developed great expertise in epidemiology. The agency remains a central repository of data and analytical talent. It continues to nurture some of the best epidemiological and medical research of the postwar period. This body of work is its central legacy and its best claim to excellence.

Notes

1. *Report of the National Academy of Sciences, National Research Council, Fiscal Year 1945–46.* Washington, D.C.: U.S. Government Printing Office, 1947, p. 52.
2. "Report of Activities of the Division of Medical Sciences, February and March, 1946," April 3, 1946, Division of Medical Sciences Files (DMS), National Academy of Sciences (NAS) Archives, Washington, D.C.
3. "Conference on Postwar Research," April 18, 1946, Committee on Veterans Medical Problems (CVMP) Files, DMS Files, NAS Archives.
4. Michael DeBakey to Norman Kirk, March 5, 1946, reprinted in "Conference on Postwar Research," NAS Archives.
5. Gilbert Beebe's discussion before the National Research Council (NRC) Division of Medical Sciences Executive Committee, April 1972, pp. 93–94, describes Harvey Cushing's failed effort after World War I to follow up head wounds in that war; DMS Files, NAS Archives.
6. "Conference on Postwar Research," April 5, 1946.
7. Committee on Veterans' Medical Problems, "Minutes of Meeting," May 7, 1946, CVMP Files, NAS Archives.
8. Committee on Veterans Medical Problems, "Draft of a Report on the Value and Feasibility of a Long-Term Research Program of Follow-up Study," June 13, 1946, p. 2, CVMP Files, NAS Archives.
9. Committee on Veterans Medical Problems, "Minutes of Meeting", May 7, 1946.
10. "Draft of a Report," June 13, 1946, pp. 2–4.
11. Paul Hawley to Frank Jewett, June 8, 1946, CVMP Files, NAS Archives; "Draft of a Report," p. 4.
12. "Draft of a Report," June 13, 1946, p. 6.
13. *Ibid.,* pp. 15, 54–55.
14. Committee on Veterans' Medical Problems, "Minutes of Meeting," June 13, 1946, CVMP Files, NAS Archives.
15. Frank Jewett to Ross Harrison and Lewis Weed, June 14, 1946; Paul Hawley to Jewett, June 8, 1946; and Jewett to Hawley, June 21, 1946, all in CVMP Files, NAS Archives. (Somewhere in the discussions, the apostrophe after "Veterans" was dropped.)

16. Lewis Weed to Detlev Bronk, August 8, 1946, and Weed to O.H. Perry Pepper, August 8, 1946, CVMP Files, NAS Archives.
17. Committee on Veterans Medical Problems, "Minutes of Meeting," September 20, 1946, CVMP Files, NAS Archives.
18. Division of Medical Sciences, Annual Report, June 30, 1965, DMS Files, NAS Archives.
19. "Minutes of Conference on Access to Medical Records of Members and Former Members of the Armed Forces," November 12, 1946, CVMP Files, NAS Archives.
20. "Draft of Report of the Chairman of the Division of Medical Sciences for the monthly meeting of the Executive Committee," December 20, 1946, DMS Files, NAS Archives.
21. Committee on Veterans Medical Problems, "Minutes of Meeting," March 14, 1967, CVMP Files, NAS Archives.
22. E.H. Cushing, acting assistant medical director for research and education, to Lewis Weed, August 19, 1947, CVMP Files, NAS Archives.
23. Subcommittee on Administrative Policies to Members of the Committee on Veterans Medical Problems, September 15, 1947, CVMP Files, NAS Archives.
24. O.H. Perry Pepper, chairman, Committee on Veterans Medical Problems, November 12, 1947, CVMP Files, NAS Archives.
25. Committee on Veterans Medical Problems, "A Report to the Chairman, Division of Medical Sciences," March 31, 1947, CVMP Files, NAS Archives.
26. Committee on Veterans Medical Problems, "Minutes of Meeting," December 11, 1947, CVMP Files, NAS Archives.
27. Committee on Veterans Medical Problems, "A Report to the Chairman, Division of Medical Sciences," March 31, 1948; "Report of the Chairman, Division of Medical Sciences," February 28, 1948, both in DMS Files, NAS Archives.
28. Committee on Veterans Medical Problems, "Minutes of Meeting," April 30, 1948, CVMP Files, NAS Archives.
29. Committee on Veterans Medical Problems, "Minutes of Meeting," October 7, 1948, CVMP Files, NAS Archives.
30. Division of Medical Sciences, "Materials for Annual Meeting," April 30, 1949, DMS Files, NAS Archives; O.H. Perry Pepper to E.H. Cushing, October 7, 1949, CVMP Files, NAS Archives.
31. O.H. Perry Pepper to E.H. Cushing, October 7, 1949.
32. "Pilot Study to Determine the Feasibility and Costs of a Mass Statistical Follow-up Program," November 12, 1948, CVMP Files, NAS Archives.
33. Committee on Veterans Medical Problems, "Minutes of Meeting," December 7, 1948, CVMP Files, NAS Archives.
34. Committee on Veterans Medical Problems, "Minutes of Meeting," January 27, 1949, CVMP Files, NAS Archives.
35. "Notes for Annual Meeting," April 30, 1949.
36. "A Report to the Chairman, Division of Medical Sciences," March 31, 1950, CVMP Files, NAS Archives.
37. Committee on Veterans Medical Problems, "Minutes of Meeting," June 11, 1949.
38. Committee on Veterans Medical Problems, "Minutes of Meeting," June 1, 1950, CVMP Files, NAS Archives.
39. Committee on Veterans Medical Problems, "Minutes of Meeting," October 9, 1950, CVMP Files, NAS Archives.
40. Committee on Veterans Medical Problems, "Report to the Division of Medical Sciences," April 30, 1951, CVMP Files, NAS Archives.
41. Wilbert Davison to Milton Winternitz, January 22, 1951, CVMP Files, NAS Archives.
42. "Report to the Division of Medical Science," April 30, 1951.

43. Herbert Marks to Milton Winternitz, January 29, 1951, and Michael DeBakey to Winternitz, January 24, 1951, CVMP Files, NAS Archives.
44. Committee on Veterans Medical Problems, "Minutes of Meeting," February 23, 1951, CVMP Files, NAS Archives.
45. "Report to the Division of Medical Sciences," April 30, 1951.
46. Gilbert Beebe, "Medical Records and the Army, Navy, and Veterans Administration Follow-up Program," February 19, 1951, Medical Follow-up Agency (MFUA) Office Files, Washington, D.C.
47. "Draft of Follow-up Section of Annual Report," April 12, 1952, CVMP Files, NAS Archives; Division of Medical Sciences, "Minutes of Annual Meeting," May 24, 1952, DMS Files, NAS Archives.
48. Committee on Veterans Medical Problems, "Minutes of Meeting," June 5, 1952, CVMP Files, NAS Archives.
49. Committee on Veterans Medical Problems, "Minutes of Meeting," December 5, 1952, NAS Archives.
50. *Report of the National Academy of Sciences: National Research Council, Fiscal Year 1951–52.* Washington, D.C.: U.S. Government Printing Office, 1955, p. 79.
51. Division of Medical Sciences, "Agenda and Minutes of Executive Committee," February 6, 1953, DMS Files, NAS Archives.
52. Bernard Cohen, Gilbert Beebe, and Seymour Jablon, "Report to the CVMP of Record Follow-up Studies," March 15, 1953, and Bernard Cohen, "Methodology of Record Follow-up Studies on Veterans," presented at American Public Health Association meeting, Cleveland, Ohio, October 24, 1952, both in MFUA Office Files. In later POW studies, however, mortality rates tended to even out (Beebe to Brian MacMahon, March 12, 1969, Committee on Epidemiology and Veterans Follow-up Studies Files, DMS Files, NAS Archives).
53. Donald Mainland, "The VA–NRC Program of Medical Follow-up Studies: Evaluations and Suggestions," March 22, 1953, DMS Files, NAS Archives.
54. Committee on Veterans Medical Problems "Minutes of Meeting," April 6, 1953, CVMP Files, NAS Archives.
55. Executive Committee, Division of Medical Sciences, "Minutes of Thirteenth Meeting," May 1, 1953, DMS Files, NAS Archives.
56. Division of Medical Sciences, "Minutes of Annual Meeting," May 23, 1953, DMS Files, NAS Archives.
57. "Dr. Cannan's Attitude Toward VA–NRC Follow-up Program," June 30, 1953, MFUA Office Files.
58. Executive Committee, Division of Medical Sciences, "Agenda" October 10, 1953, DMS Files, NAS Archives.
59. Executive Committee, Division of Medical Sciences, "Minutes of Fourteenth Meeting," October 10, 1953, DMS Files, NAS Archives.
60. "The Chairman's News Letter," November 1953, DMS Files, NAS Archives.
61. Committee on Veterans Medical Problems, "Minutes of Meeting," December 7, 1953, CVMP Files, NAS Archives.
62. "The NRC Program of Medical Follow-up Studies," December 21, 1953, DMS Files, NAS Archives.
63. Executive Committee, Division of Medical Sciences, "Minutes of Fifteenth Meeting," January 18, 1954, DMS Files, NAS Archives.
64. Keith Cannan to William Rubey, chairman, National Research Council, March 22, 1954, DMS Files, NAS Archives; "The Chairman's News Letter," March 1954, DMS Files, NAS Archives.
65. See publications: VA Multiple Sclerosis Study Group. Isoniazid in the treatment of multiple sclerosis: Report on VA Cooperative Study. *Trans. Am. Neurol. Assoc.* 128–131, 1956; Isoniazid in the treatment of multiple sclerosis, *JAMA* 163:168–172, 1957.

66. "Recent Development in the NRC Program of Medical Follow-up Studies," November 12, 1954, DMS Files, NAS Archives. Rheumatic fever research: Engleman, E.P., Hollister, L.E., Klob, F.O. Sequelae of rheumatic fever in men: Four to eight year follow-up study *JAMA* 155: 1134–1140, 1954. World War II prisoner of war research: Cohen, B.M., Cooper, M.Z. *A Follow-up Study of World War II Prisoners of War.* VA Medical Monograph. Washington, D.C.: U.S. Government Printing Office, 1955.

67. Executive Committee, Division of Medical Sciences, "Minutes of Seventeenth Meeting," November 29, 1954, DMS Files, NAS Archives.

68. Division of Medical Sciences, "Annual Report, 1953–1954," mimeo, DMS Files, NAS Archives.

69. "Basis for Inter-Agency Memorandum of Understanding in Regard to Medical Follow-up Studies," MFUA Office Files.

70. Division of Medical Sciences, "Executive Committee Agenda," May 20, 1955, DMS Files, NAS Archives.

71. "Fiscal Year 1956 Budget of Follow-up Agency," October 4, 1955, DMS Files, NAS Archives.

72. "Fiscal Year 1956 Program of the Follow-up Agency," October 4, 1955, DMS Files, NAS Archives.

73. Committee on Veterans Medical Problems, "Minutes of 33rd Meeting," March 30, 1957, CVMP Files, NAS Archives.

74. Committee on Veterans Medical Problems, "Minutes of 32nd Meeting," June 15, 1956, CVMP Files, NAS Archives.

75. James Neel, MD to Bernard Cohen, May 2, 1956, CVMP Files, NAS Archives.

76. Ad Hoc Committee on Studies of Veteran Twins, "Minutes of First Meeting," February 21, 1957, DMS Files, NAS Archives.

77. Committee on Veterans Medical Problems, "Minutes of 33rd Meeting," March 30, 1957, CVMP Files, NAS Archives.

78. Committee on Veterans Medical Problems, "Minutes of 34th Meeting," December 9, 1957, CVMP Files, NAS Archives.

79. Gilbert Beebe, "Medical Follow-up Studies Based on Military Experience," paper before the Society of Medical Consultants to the Armed Forces, November 11, 1957, DMS Files, NAS Archives.

80. Division of Medical Sciences, "Annual Report," 1 July 1956–30 June 1957, DMS Files, NAS Archives.

81. Division of Medical Sciences, "Annual Report," fiscal year 1958, DMS Files, NAS Archives.

82. Gilbert Beebe to Lyndon Lee, November 14, 1960, DMS Files, NAS Archives.

83. *Annual Report, National Academy of Sciences, National Research Council, Fiscal Year 1958–1959.* Washington, D.C.: U.S. Government Printing Office, 1960, p. 67.

84. "Medical Genetic Studies of Veteran Twins," February 19, 1959, CVMP Files, NAS Archives.

85. Committee on Veterans Medical Problems, "Minutes of 36th Meeting," April 11, 1959, CVMP Files, NAS Archives.

86. "Annual Report of Follow-up Agency," July 11, 1960, CVMP Files, NAS Archives.

87. Keith Cannan to William Middleton, May 11, 1961, CVMP Files, NAS Archives.

88. Gilbert Beebe to Committee on Veterans Medical Problems, January 23, 1961, CVMP Files, NAS Archives.

89. Committee on Veterans Medical Problems, "Minutes of Thirty-Eighth Meeting," February 15, 1961, CVMP Files, NAS Archives.

90. Henry Brosin to Walter Barton, December 4, 1961; Thomas Chalmers to Dean Nefzger, December 7, 1961; Gilbert Beebe to Keith Cannan, December 26, 1961, all in DMS Files, NAS Archives.

91. Keith Cannan to the Record, January 18, 1962, DMS Files, NAS Archives.

92. Division of Medical Sciences, "Annual Report, 1 July 1960–30 June 1961," DMS Files, NAS Archives.

93. "Program of Medical Follow-up Studies on Veterans," May 31, 1962, DMS Files, NAS Archives; Gilbert Beebe to staff members, Division of Medical Sciences, March 7, 1962, MFUA Office Files.

94. Thomas Francis to Gilbert Beebe, May 17, 1962; James Neel to Beebe, May 21, 1962; and Beebe to Keith Cannan, June 8, 1962, all in DMS Files, NAS Archives.

95. Keith Cannan to Michael DeBakey, July 3, 1962; Cannan to William Stone, September 19, 1962; Esmond Long to Cannan, September 27, 1962; Gordon Scott to Cannon, October 1, 1962; Fred Hodges to Cannan, October 3, 1962; and Donald Mainland to Cannan, October 19, 1962, all in DMS Files, NAS Archives.

96. Division of Medical Sciences, "Minutes of Annual Meeting," April 9, 1963, DMS Files, NAS Archives.

97. "Annual Report of the Follow-up Agency," July 18, 1963, DMS Files, NAS Archives.

98. "Annual Report of the Follow-up Agency," July 17, 1964, DMS Files, NAS Archives.

99. Gilbert Beebe to Keith Cannan, October 15, 1964, and Division of Medical Sciences Annual Report, June 30, 1970, both in DMS Files, NAS Archives.

100. Keith Cannan to Thomas Francis, Jr., December 16, 1964, DMS Files, NAS Archives.

101. Keith Cannan to Brian MacMahon, April 6, 1965, Committee on Epidemiology and Veterans Follow-up Studies (CEVFUS) Files, NAS Archives.

102. Brian MacMahon to Keith Cannan, April 9, 1965, CEVFUS Files, NAS Archives.

103. Keith Cannan to Michael DeBakey, July 13, 1965, CEVFUS Files, NAS Archives.

104. Keith Cannan to Williams Jordan, University of Virginia School of Medicine, July 13, 1965, and Cannan to Paul Lemkau, Johns Hopkins School of Hygiene and Public Health, July 13, 1965, both in CEVFUS Files, NAS Archives. Similar letters went out to the rest of the new committee.

105. Gilbert Beebe memo to Keith Cannan, "Recommendation for Membership of New Committee to Guide Program of Medical Follow-up Studies on Veterans," May 28, 1965, CEVFUS Files, NAS Archives.

106. "Essential Aspects of the Program of Medical Follow-up Studies on Veterans," November 8, 1965, CEVFUS Files, NAS Archives.

107. "Annual Report of the Follow-up Agency," June 1965, DMS Files, NAS Archives.

108. Minutes, CEVFUS Meeting, November 26, 1965, CEVFUS Files, NAS Archives; *Annual Report of the National Academy of Sciences, Fiscal Year 1964–1965.* Washington, D.C.: U.S. Government Printing Office, 1967.

109. Minutes, CEVFUS Meeting, March 18, 1966, CEVFUS Files, NAS Archives.

110. "Annual Report of the Follow-up Agency," June 15, 1966, CEVFUS Files, NAS Archives.

111. A. Hiram Simon memo to Gilbert Beebe, "Roster 517, loss of part of file," June 21, 1965, R-4 Files, MFUA Office Files.

112. Dean Nefzger to Gilbert Beebe, May 11, 1967; Beebe to Nefzger, May 16, 1967; Nefzger to Ida C. Merriam, Social Security Administration, July 17, 1967; Merriam to Nefzger, July 19, 1967; and Lenore A. Epstein, Social Security Administration to Nefzger, August 23, 1967, all in R-4 Files, MFUA Office Files. The wording of the latter suggests that a more "politically wired" organization might have been able to maneuver a less direct way around the confidentiality issue and receive the necessary information. On veterans organizations: Nefzger memo to CEVFUS, "Use of Veteran Service Organizations for Field Work in POW Study," May 1, 1968, CEVFUS Files, NAS Archives.

113. Arthur A. Bressi, national commander, American Defenders of Bataan and Corregidor, Inc., to Brian MacMahon, August 1, 1966, and Seymour Jablon to Bressi, August 5, 1966, both in R-4 Files, MFUA Office Files; Gilbert Beebe to MacMahon, April 7, 1969, CEVFUS Files, NAS Archives.

114. Minutes, CEVFUS Meeting, April 27, 1967, CEVFUS Files, NAS Archives; Seymour Jablon to Leopold M. Macari, Veterans Administration, June 10, 1966, R-19 Files, MFUA Office Files. The paper was published as Jablon, S., Neel, J.V., Gershowitz, H., Atkinson, G.F. The

NAS–NRC Twin Panel: Methods of construction of the panel, zygosity diagnosis, and proposed use. *American Journal of Human Genetics*, 19:133–161, 1967.

115. Minutes, CEVFUS Meeting, March 18, 1966, CEVFUS Files, NAS Archives.

116. *Ibid.* Also James Neel to Gilbert Beebe, May 12, 1969, CEVFUS Files, NAS Archives.

117. Minutes, CEVFUS Meeting, April 27, 1967, CEVFUS Files, NAS Archives, and Seymour Jablon, "Uses of the Roster of Veteran Twins," appendix to Division of Medical Sciences Annual Meeting Minutes, March 13, 1967, DMS Files, NAS Archives.

118. Minutes, CEVFUS Meeting, May 23, 1968, CEVFUS Files, NAS Archives.

119. Seymour Jablon to Brian MacMahon, June 19, 1967, and MacMahon to Jablon, July 6, 1967, both CEVFUS Files, NAS Archives. Division of Medical Sciences, Annual Report, June 30, 1969, DMS Files, NAS Archives.

120. Division of Medical Sciences, "Minutes of Annual Meeting," March 13, 1967, DMS Files, NAS Archives; "Annual Report of Follow-up Agency," June 26, 1967, CEVFUS Files, NAS Archives.

121. Brian MacMahon to Robert Q. Marston, director of the National Institutes of Health, December 23, 1968, and Gilbert Beebe to MacMahon, July 8, 1969, both in CEVFUS Files, NAS Archives.

122. "Annual Report of the Follow-up Agency," June 17, 1968, CEVFUS Files; Division of Medical Sciences, "Minutes of Annual Meeting," March 11, 1968, DMS Files, both in NAS Archives.

123. "Minutes of the Meeting of Subcommittee on Twin Studies, Washington, D.C., 9 November 1969" (Zdenek Hrubec), "Status of the NRC Twin Registry Activities," November 21, 1969, and Gilbert Beebe to Ransom J. Arthur, August 18, 1970, all in CEVFUS Files, NAS Archives.

124. Division of Medical Sciences, "Annual Report," June 30, 1969, DMS Files; "Long-Term Commitments," Item V-C in December 1969 CEVFUS Agenda Book, CEVFUS Files, both in NAS Archives.

125. Robert J. Keehn and A.H. Simon (MFUA staff members), memo to Gilbert Beebe, "AEC Support for FUA," December 10, 1969; Beebe to Richard Remington, University of Texas, December 22, 1969; and Beebe to Ransom J. Arthur, August 18, 1970, all in CEVFUS Files, NAS Archives. Also Beebe's discussion of the Atomic Bomb Casualty Commission (ABCC) arrangement before the DMS Executive Committee, April 1972, DMS Files, NAS Archives.

126. Division of Medical Sciences, "Annual Report," June 30, 1970, DMS Files, NAS Archives.

127. Charles Dunham, Division of Medical Sciences, to Rear Admiral Frank V. Voris, U.S. Navy, December 23, 1968, and Voris to Dunham, March 17, 1969, both in CEVFUS Files, NAS Archives.

128. Minutes, CEVFUS Meeting, May 1, 1969, and Brian MacMahon to Ransom J. Arthur, University of California Medical School, December 1, 1970, both in CEVFUS Files, NAS Archives.

129. Gilbert Beebe to Julius Sendroy, Jr., National Naval Medical Center, December 17, 1969, CEVFUS Files, NAS Archives.

130. Gilbert Beebe to Ransom J. Arthur, October 22, 1970, CEVFUS Files, NAS Archives.

131. Gilbert Beebe to Colonel John White, Marine Corps, January 14, 1971, and Michael Beebe to DeBakey, April 30, 1971, both in CEVFUS Files, NAS Archives.

132. Gilbert Beebe to Richard Remington, December 22, 1969, and Beebe to Ransom J. Arthur, August 18, 1970, both in CEVFUS Files, NAS Archives.

133. Gilbert Beebe to Stuart Roberts, Peoria School of Medicine, June 4, 1973, and John F. Stremple, Pittsburgh VA Hospital, to Michael DeBakey, March 7, 1977, both in CEVFUS Files, NAS Archives.

134. Division of Medical Sciences, "Annual Report," June 30, 1971, DMS Files, NAS Archives; Minutes, CEVFUS Meeting, May 17, 1971, and Charles Dunham to Brig. General Richard R. Taylor, U.S. Army, June 9, 1971, both in CEVFUS Files, NAS Archives.

135. Gilbert Beebe to Gordon Allen, NIMH, May 22, 1970, and Beebe to file, "Discussion with Dr.

Lyndon Lee, 17 March 1971 in re Membership of Committee on Epidemiology and Veterans Follow-up Studies," March 22, 1971, both in CEVFUS Files, NAS Archives.

136. Gilbert Beebe to Charles Dunham, March 22, 1971, CEVFUS Files, NAS Archives.

137. Minutes, CEVFUS Meeting, May 17, 1971, CEVFUS Files, NAS Archives.

138. "Recommendations to the Research Service, VA Department of Medicine and Surgery Concerning Support of the Activities of the Follow-up Agency at National Research Council–National Academy of Sciences," Lawrence W. Shaw and Armand Littman, February 16, 1972, CEVFUS Files, NAS Archives.

139. Gilbert Beebe to Frederick H. Epstein, University of Michigan, May 2, 1972, CEVFUS Files, NAS Archives; Beebe discussion with the DMS Executive Committee, April 1972, DMS Files, NAS Archives. The study is Beebe memo to file, "Source of Investigation Interest in R-Projects," March 31, 1977, CEVFUS Files, NAS Archives.

140. Gilbert Beebe to William J. Zukel, National Heart and Lung Institute (NHLI), June 2, 1972, and Beebe to Brian MacMahon, March 6, 1972, both in CEVFUS Files, NAS Archives.

141. *Ibid.*

142. Division of Medical Sciences, "Annual Report," June 30, 1972, and Division of Medical Sciences, "Annual Report," June 30, 1973, both in DMS Files, NAS Archives; Minutes, CEVFUS Meeting, April 11, 1972; Charles Dunham to Robert McClelland, University of Texas, July 24, 1972; and Gilbert Beebe to Dunham, May 28, 1971, all in CEVFUS Files, NAS Archives.

143. Gilbert Beebe, discussion before the DMS Executive Committee, April 1972, and Division of Medical Sciences Annual Report, June 1972, both in DMS Files, NAS Archives; "Report of Progress . . . Medical Follow-up and Epidemiologic Studies on Veterans," February 29, 1972, CEVFUS Files, NAS Archives.

144. Charles Dunham to Brian MacMahon, July 24, 1972, and Gilbert Beebe memo to file "Conference with Dr. Lee, VACO, Relative to the FUA Program and VA Support, 26 March 1970," both in CEVFUS Files, NAS Archives.

145. Minutes, CEVFUS Meeting, January 11, 1973, and "Service by the Follow-up Agency to Other Investigators," December 26, 1972," both in CEVFUS Files, NAS Archives.

146. Gilbert Beebe to CEVFUS, July 23, 1973, "Fire Losses at St. Louis Records Center" (apparently authored by Seymour Jablon), May 9, 1974, and Minutes, CEVFUS Meeting, May 21, 1974, all in CEVFUS Files, NAS Archives.

147. Minutes, CEVFUS Meeting, June 15, 1973; Seymour Jablon to Richard Remington, September 11, 1973; and Gilbert Beebe to Frederick H. Epstein, July 26, 1973, all in CEVFUS Files, NAS Archives.

148. Minutes, CEVFUS Meeting, February 7, 1975, CEVFUS Files, NAS Archives.

149. Gilbert Beebe to Stuart Roberts, Peoria School of Medicine, June 4, 1973; Beebe to Seymour Jablon, August 20, 1973; and Beebe to Capt. Ransom J. Arthur, Navy Medical Neuropsychiatric Research Unit, January 22, 1973, all in CEVFUS Files, NAS Archives.

150. "Report of Progress . . . Medical Follow-up and Epidemiologic Studies on Veterans," February 26, 1973, CEVFUS Files, NAS Archives.

151. Minutes, CEVFUS Meeting, May 21, 1974; Seymour Jablon to Richard Remington, June 11, 1974; and Remington to Thomas Newcomb, Veterans Administration, August 22, 1974, all in CEVFUS Files, NAS Archives.

152. "Proposal to Create Magnetic Tape Index to Navy Hospital Diagnoses in World War II (1944–1945)" (Seymour Jablon), May 11, 1976, and Minutes, CEVFUS Meeting, May 11, 1983, both in CEVFUS Files, NAS Archives.

153. *Ibid.* Taubman's research resulted in three journal publications: Taubman, P. The determinants of earnings: Genetics, family and other environments: A study of white male twins. *American Economic Review* 66:858–870, 1976; Earnings, education, genetics, and environment. *Journal of Human Resources* 11(fall):447–461, 1976; and What we learn from estimating the genetic

contribution to inequality of earning: Reply. *American Economic Review* 68:970–976, 1978. This research also resulted in a book chapter: Behrman, J., Taubman, P., Wales, T. Controlling for and measuring the effects of genetics and family environment in equations for schooling and labor market success. In (P. Taubman ed.): *Kinometrics: Determinant of Socioeconomic Success Within and Between Families*. New York: North-Holland Publishing Company, 1977.

154. *Ibid.*

155. Gilbert Beebe memo to CEVFUS, "Future Program," May 10, 1976, CEVFUS Files, NAS Archives.

156. Philip Handler, NAS president, to Carole W. Parsons, executive director, Privacy Protection Study Commission, May 27, 1976, with attachment "Some Implications of the 1974 Privacy Act, and of the Extension of Its Principles to Health-Care Institutions, for Biomedical Research," MFUA Office Files.

157. Gilbert Beebe to James Neel, March 23, 1976, and Minutes, CEVFUS Meetings, May 25, 1976, and December 15, 1976, all in CEVFUS Files, NAS Archives.

158. Seymour Jablon to Richard Remington, October 8, 1976, CEVFUS Files; Alvin G. Lazen, Assembly of Life Sciences, to Paul Marks, Columbia University, November 8, 1976, Accession 91-028-02/11; Gilbert Beebe to Remington, March 29, 1977, CEVFUS Files; Beebe to CEVFUS, March 31, 1977, Accession 91-028-02/11; Remington to CEVFUS, March 31, 1977, Accession 91-028-02/11; and Councilman Morgan to Paul Ebert, Mark Hegsted, Brian MacMahon, Richard Remington, and Donald Seldin, April 18, 1977, Accession 91-028-02/11, all in NAS Archives.

159. "Report of the Subcommittee on Epidemiological Studies of Cardiovascular Disease" (Reuel Stallones), December 1976, and Minutes, CEVFUS Meeting, December 15, 1976, both in CEVFUS Files, NAS Archives.

160. "Bibliography of the Medical Follow-up Agency," September 1998, MFUA unpublished document.

161. "Critical Issues for the Future," Item VI, CEVFUS Meeting (April 11–12, 1977) Agenda, March 30, 1977, CEVFUS Files, NAS Archives.

162. Zdenek Hrubec to Richard Remington, April 1, 1977, and Minutes, CEVFUS Meetings, April 11–12, 1977, and March 15, 1979, all in CEVFUS Files, NAS Archives.

163. Barbara S. Hulka, University of North Carolina at Chapel Hill, to Seymour Jablon, July 16, 1981, and Jablon to Alvin Lazen, "Your Draft Letter to Brian MacMahon Dated 10/25/82" (letter to MacMahon enclosed), MFUA Office Files. MacMahon at the time had returned to the CEVFUS chair.

164. Minutes, CEVFUS Meeting, May 11, 1983, MFUA Office Files.

165. *Ibid.*

166. Seymour Jablon to CEVFUS; April 3, 1978; Smith, R.J. Study of atomic veterans fuels controversy. *Science* 221(4612):733–4, 1983; and Anderson, C. NAS to redo atomic studies found to be flawed. *Nature* 359:354, 1992.

167. Robinette, C.D. Cancer among atomic veterans: No consistent increase found, but excess leukemia confirmed in one group. *CLS Lifelines* 11(2–3):5, 1985; Seymour Jablon to Kenneth I. Shine, president, Institute of Medicine, January 27, 1993, MFUA Office Files.

168. C. Dennis Robinette, MFUA staff, to Richard Remington, July 29, 1985; Seymour Jablon to Remington, November 4, 1985; Minutes, CEVFUS Meeting, November 13, 1985; and Robinette to Remington, March 10, 1986, all in MFUA Office Files.

169. Minutes, CEVFUS Meeting, November 13, 1985, MFUA Office Files.

170. Richard Remington to Seymour Jablon, March 3, 1986, and C. Dennis Robinette to Remington, March 10, 1986, both in MFUA Office Files. (This HIV study was one of the first that the MFUA presented in 1988 to its new parent body, the Institute of Medicine, for review.)

171. "Report of an Ad Hoc Executive Committee charged to review the Medical Follow-up Agency" (MacMahon committee), July 27, 1987, Accession 91-028-02/11, NAS Archives.

172. Alvin Lazen, Commission on Life Sciences (CLS) executive director, to MFUA staff, June 13, 1987, and John Dowling, CLS chairman to Brian MacMahon, August 14, 1987; and William Page to Richard Remington, October 6, 1987, both from Accession 91-028-02/11, NAS Archives; the latter is from MFUA Office Files.

173. Gilbert Beebe to Frank Press, NAS president, June 19, 1987, and Beebe memo to Records "Discussion with Staff of Senate Committee on Veterans Affairs Concerning the Status of the Medical Follow-up Agency of the National Research Council," August 7, 1987, both from the MFUA office files; William Page to Alvin Lazen, November 5, 1987, and Commission of Life Sciences "Status Report" on Follow-up to MFUA Review, December 10–11, 1987, both from Accession 91-028-02/11, NAS Archives.

174. Medical Follow-up Agency, "Annual Report," December 31, 1986, Accession 91-028-02/11, NAS Archives; National Research Council, Commission on Life Sciences, Medical Follow-up Agency, June 4, 1987, and Minutes, CEVFUS Meeting, June 4, 1987, both from MFUA Office Files.

175. Office of Technology Assessment, "Report of an OTA Workshop on the Medical Follow-up Agency," November 1988, MFUA Office Files.

176. Richard B. Setlow, Brookhaven National Laboratory, to John Dowling, Harvard University, May 6, 1988; William Page to Michael DeBakey, May 24, 1988; and Page to DeBakey, June 29, 1988, all in MFUA Office Files.

177. O. Dale Williams and C. Morton Hawkins, "Report of the Site Visit to the Medical Follow-up Agency of the Institute of Medicine," 1989, MFUA Office Files.

178. William Page to Samuel Thier, IOM president, December 29, 1989; Page to Richard Remington, January 5, 1990; and Edward J. Derwinski, Secretary of Veterans Affairs, to Senator Alan Cranston, Senate Veterans Affairs Committee, May 4, 1990, all in MFUA Office Files.

179. Minutes, CEVFUS Meeting, May 21, 1990, MFUA Office Files.

180. Minutes, CEVFUS Meeting, September 24, 1991, MFUA Office Files.

181. Chris Howson, MFUA interim director, to CEVFUS, May 11, 1993; and Dick Miller, MFUA director, to Ken Shine, IOM president, July 23, 1993, both in MFUA Office Files. Also interview with Dick Miller, May 28, 1998.

Medical Follow-up Agency Publication List, 1946–1996

1946

National Research Council, Division of Medical Sciences. Report on the Value and Feasibility of a Long-Term Program of Follow-up Study and Clinical Research. Washington, D.C.: 1946.

1949

Allam, M.W., Nulsen, F.E., Lewey, F.H. Electrical intraneural biopolar stimulation of peripheral nerves in the dog. *J. Am. Vet. Med. Assoc.* 114:87–89, 1949.

Bender, M.B., Teuber, H.L. Disturbances in visual perception following cerebral lesions. *Psychol.* 28:223–233, 1949.

Bender, M.B., Teuber, H.L. Psychopathology of vision. Pp. 163–192 in *Progress in Neurology and Psychiatry*. New York: Grune and Stratton, 1949.

Freeman, N.E., Fullenlove, T.M., Wylie, E.J., Gilfillan, R.S. The Valsalva Maneuver: An aid for the contrast visualization of the aorta and great vessels. *Ann. Surg.* 130(Sept.):398–416, 1949.

Lewey, F.H. Quantitative examination of sensibility in peripheral nerve injuries. *Confin. Neurol.* 9:206–210, 1949.

Lewey, F.H., Nulsen, F.E. Management and assessment of peripheral nerve injuries. *J. Ins. Med.* 4(July):31–33, 1949.

Teuber, H.L., Bender, M.D. Alterations in pattern vision following trauma of occipital lobes in man. *J. Gen. Psychol.* 40(Jan.):37–57, 1949.

1950

Bender, M.B., Teuber, H.L., Battersby, W.S. Discrimination of weights by men with penetrating lesions of parietal lobes. *Trans. Am. Neurol. Assoc.* 75:252–255, 1950.

Davis, C.H., Woodhall, B. Changes in the arteriae nervorum in peripheral nerve injuries in man. *J. Neuropathol. Exp. Neurol.* 9 July:335–343, 1950.

Friedman, M. Tumors of the testis and their treatment. Pp. 276–308 in U.V. Portmann (ed.), *Clinical Therapeutic Radiology.* New York: Nelson, 1950.

Herz, E., Yahr, M.D. Painful sensory syndrome during nerve regeneration. *Trans. Am. Neurol. Assoc.* 75 (June):213–218, 1950.

Michael, M., Jr. The course of sarcoidosis as influenced by cortisone. Pp. 85–86 in *Proceedings of the VA Conference on Cortisone Research,* August 15–16, 1950.

Michael, M., Jr., Cole, R.M., Beeson, P.B., Olson, B.J. Sarcoidosis: Preliminary report on study of 350 cases with special reference to epidemiology. *Am. Rev. Tuberc.* 62 (Oct.):403–407, 1950.

Michael, M., Jr., Cole, R.M., Beeson, P.B., Olson, B.J. Sarcoidosis: Preliminary observations from an analysis of 350 cases. *Natl. Tuberc. Assoc.* 46:208–212, 1950.

Pepper, O.H.P. Medical follow-up studies of veterans. *Trans. Assoc. Life Ins. Med. Dir. Am.* 33:99–111, 1950.

Teuber, H.L. Neuropsychology. Pp 30–52 in R.E. Harris, et al. (eds.) *Recent advances in diagnostic psychological testing: A Critical Summary.* Springfield, Ill.: Charles C. Thomas, 1950.

Teuber, H.L., Bender, M.B. Perception of apparent movement across acquired scotomata in the visual field. *Am. Psychol.* 5 (July):271–272, 1950.

Yahr, M.D., Herz, E., Moldaver, J., Grundfest, H. Electromyographic patterns in reinnervated muscle. *Arch. Neurol. Psychiatry* 63 (May):728–738, 1950.

Zieve, L., Hill, E., Nesbitt, S. Studies of liver function tests. I. A combined intravenous bromsulfalein-hippuric acid-galactose test. *J. Lab. Clin. Med.* 36(Nov.):705–709, 1950.

1951

Amory, H.I., Brick, I.B. Irradiation damage of the intestines following 1,000-kV. Roentgen therapy. Evaluation of tolerance dose. *Radiology* 56(Jan):49–57, 1951.

Auerbach, O., Friedman, M., Weiss, L., Amory, H.I. Extraskeletal osteogenic sarcoma arising in irradiated tissue. *Cancer* 4 (Sept.):1095–1106, 1951.

Battersby, W.S. The regional gradient of critical flicker frequency after frontal or occipital lobe injury. *J. Exp. Psychol.* 42 (July):59–68, 1951.

Battersby, W.S., Bender, M.B., Teuber, H.L. Effects of total light flux on critical flicker frequency after frontal lobe lesion. *J. Exp. Psychol.* 42(Aug):135–142, 1951.

Beebe, G.W. Medical Records and the Army, Navy and Veterans Administration Follow-up Program. Military Medicine Notes, Army Medical Service Graduate School, Washington, D.C., Vol. 1, Section A, 1951.

Bender, M.B., Krieger, H.P. Visual function in perimetrically blind fields. *Arch. Neurol. Psychiatry* 65(Jan.):72–79, 1951.

Bender, M.B., Teuber, H.L., Battersby, W.S. Visual field defects after gunshot wounds of higher visual pathways. *Trans. Am. Neurol. Assoc.* 76:192–194, 1951.

Brill, N.Q., Beebe, G.W. Follow-up study of psychoneuroses: Preliminary report. *Am. J. Psychiatry* 108(Dec.):417–425, 1951.

Freni, D.R., Warren, R. End-results of rehabilitation of war wounds of the hand. *Arch. Surg.* 63(Dec.):774–782, 1951.

Jaffe, R. Influence of cerebral trauma on kinesthetic after-effects. *Am. Psychol.* 6(July):265(July), 1951.

Krieger, H.P., Bender, M.B. Dark adaptation in peri-metrically blind fields. *Arch. Ophthalmol.* 46(Dec.):625–636, 1951.

Michael, M., Jr. The treatment of sarcoidosis with cortisone. Pp. 65-68 in *Proceedings of a Symposium on Cortisone and ACTH*. Transactions of 47th Annual Meeting, National Tuberculosis Association, 1951.

Ripley, H.S., Wolf, S. Long-term study of combat area schizophrenic reactions. *Am. J. Psychiatry* 108 (Dec.):409–416, 1951.

Schwartz, S., Zieve, L., Watson, C.J. An improved method for the determination of urinary coproporphyrin and an evaluation of factors influencing the analysis. *J. Lab. Clin. Med.* 37(June):843–859, 1951.

Teuber, H.L., Battersby, W.S., Bender, M.B. Performance of complex visual tasks after cerebral lesions. *J. Nerv. Ment. Dis.* 114(Nov.):413–429, 1951.

Teuber, H.L., Bender, M.B. Neuro-ophthalmology: The oculomotor system. *Prog. Neurol. Psychiatry* 6:148–178, 1951.

Zieve, L., Hanson, M., Hill, E. Studies of liver function tests. II. Derivation of a correction allowing use of the bromsulfalein test in jaundiced patients. *J. Lab. Clin. Med.* 37(Jan.):40–51, 1951.

Zieve, L., Hill, E., Hanson, M., Falcone, A.B., Watson, C.J. Normal and abnormal variations and clinical significance of the one-minute and total serum bilirubin determinations. *J. Lab. Clin. Med.* 38(Sept.):446–469, 1951.

1952

Bender, M.B. *Disorders in Perception with Particular Reference to the Phenomena of Extinction and Displacement*. Springfield, Ill.: Charles C. Thomas, 1952.

Brill, N.Q., Beebe, G.W. Psychoneuroses: Military applications of a follow-up study. *Armed Forces Med. Bull.* 2(Jan.):15–33, 1952.

Brill, N.Q., Beebe, G.W. Some applications of a follow-up study to psychiatric standards for mobilization. *Am. J. Psychiatry* 109(Dec.):401–420, 1952.

Dixon, F.J., Moore, R.A. Tumors of the male sex organs. Section 8. In *Atlas of Tumor Pathology*. Washington, DC: Armed Forces Institute of Pathology, 1952.

Glenn, W.W.L., Maraist, F.B., Braaten, O.M. Treatment of frostbite with particular reference to the use of adrenocorticotrophic hormone (ACTH). *N. Engl. J. Med.* 247(Aug.):191–200, 1952.

1953

Barr, J.S., Elliston, W., Musnick, H., DeLorme, T., Hanelin, J., Thibodeau, A.A. Fracture of the carpal navicular (scaphoid) bone. An end-result study in military personnel. *J. Bone Joint Surg.* 35A(July):609–624, 1953.

Battersby, W.S., Teuber, H.L., Bender, M.B. Problem solving behavior in men with frontal or occipital brain injuries. *J. Psychol.* 35(Apr.):329–351, 1953.

Brill, N.Q., Beebe, G.W., Loewenstein, R.L. Age and resistance to military stress. *U.S. Armed Forces Med. J.* 4(Sept.):1247–1266, 1953.

Cohen, B.M. Methodology of record follow-up studies on veterans. *Am. J. Public Health* 43(Oct.):1292–1298, 1953.

Dixon, F.J., Moore, R.A. Testicular tumors. A clinicopathological study. *Cancer* 6(May):427–454, 1953.

Zieve, L. Studies of liver function tests. III. Dependence of percentage cholesterol esters upon the degree of jaundice. *J. Lab. Clin. Med.* 42(July):134–139, 1953.

Zieve, L., Hanson, M. Studies of liver function tests. IV. Effect of repeated injections of sodium benzoate on the formation of hippuric acid in patients with liver disease. *J. Lab. Clin. Med.* 42(Nov.):872–876, 1953.

Zieve, L., Hill, E. Influence of alcohol consumption on hepatic function in healthy gainfully employed men. *J. Lab. Clin. Med.* 42(Nov.):705–712, 1953.

Zieve, L., Hill, E., Nesbitt, S., Zieve, B. The incidence of residuals of viral hepatitis. *Gastroenterology* 25(Dec.):495–531, 1953.

Zieve, L., Hill, E., Schwartz, S., Watson, C.J. Normal limits of urinary coproporphyrin excretion determined by an improved method. *J. Lab. Clin. Med.* 41(May):663–669, 1953.

1954

Engleman, E.P., Hollister, L.E., Kolb, F.O. Sequelae of rheumatic fever in men: four to eight year follow-up study. *JAMA* 155(July):1134–1140, 1954.

Friedman, M. Calculated risks of radiation injury of normal tissue in the treatment of cancer of the testis, Vol. 1. Pp. 390–400 in *Proceedings of the Second National Cancer Conference*, Cincinnati, Ohio, March 3–5, 1952. New York: American Cancer Society, 1954.

Ripley, H.S., Wolf, S. The course of wartime schizophrenia compared with a control group. *J. Nerv. Ment. Dis.* 120 (Sept.–Oct.):184–195, 1954.

1955

Brick, I.B. Effects of million volt irradiation on the gastrointestinal tract. *Arch. Intern. Med.* 96(July):26–31, 1955.

Cohen, B.M., Cooper, M.Z. *A Follow-up Study of World War II Prisoners of War.* VA Medical Monograph. Washington, D.C.: U.S. Government Printing Office, 1955.

Gentry, J.T., Notowsky, H.M., Michael, M. Studies on the epidemiology of sarcoidosis in the United States: The relationship to soil areas and to urban–rural residence. *J. Clin. Invest.* 34(Dec.):1839–1856, 1955.

Long, E.R., Jablon, S. *Tuberculosis in the Army of the United States in World War II.* VA Medical Monograph. Washington, D.C.: U.S. Government Printing Office, 1955.

Most, H. Treatment of schistosomiasis. *Am. J. Trop. Med. Hyg.* 4(May):455–459, 1955.

Neefe, J.R., Gambescia, J.M., Kurtz, C.H., Smith, H.D., Beebe, G.W., Jablon, S., Reinhold, J.G., Williams, S.C. Prevalence and nature of hepatic disturbance following acute viral hepatitis with jaundice. *Ann. Intern. Med.* 43(July):1–32, 1955.

Simeone, F.A. A preliminary follow-up on cases of cold injury from World War II. Pp. 197–223 in *Cold Injury, Transactions of the Fourth Conference.* New York: Josiah Macy, Jr. Foundation, 1955.

Woodhall, B. (ed.) *Preliminary Report. Peripheral Nerve Regeneration Study Centers.* Durham, N.C.: Duke Medical School and Hospital, June 1955.

Zieve, L., Hill, E. Note on hepatic function one to three decades after an episode of jaundice during childhood. *Gastroenterology* 28(Mar.):418–423, 1955.

Zieve, L., Hill, E. An evaluation of factors influencing the discriminative effectiveness of a group of liver function tests. I: The utilization of multiple measurements in medicine. *Gastroenterology* 28(May):759–765, 1955.

Zieve, L., Hill, E. An evaluation of factors influencing the discriminative effectiveness of a group of liver function tests. II: Normal limits of eleven representative hepatic tests. *Gastroenterology* 28(May):766–784, 1955.

Zieve, L., Hill, E. An evaluation of factors influencing the discriminative effectiveness of a group of liver function tests. III: Relative effectiveness of hepatic tests in cirrhosis. *Gastroenterology* 28(May):785–802, 1955.

Zieve, L., Hill, E. An evaluation of factors influencing the discriminative effectiveness of a group of liver function tests. IV: Nature of the interrelationships among hepatic tests in cirrhosis. *Gastroenterology* 28(June):914–926, 1955.

Zieve, L., Hill, E., Hanson, M. An evaluation of factors influencing the discriminative effectiveness of a group of liver function tests. V: Relative effectiveness of hepatic tests in viral hepatitis. *Gastroenterology* 28(June):927–942, 1955.

Zieve, L., Hill, E., Hanson, M. An evaluation of factors influencing the discriminative effectiveness of a group of liver function tests. VI: Nature of the interrelationships among hepatic tests in viral hepatitis. *Gastroenterology* 28(June):943–952, 1955.

1956

Brill, N.Q., Beebe, G.W. *A Follow-up Study of War Neuroses.* VA Medical Monograph. Washington, D.C.: U.S. Government Printing Office, 1956.

Friedman, M. The superior value of supervoltage irradiation in special situations: Carcinoma of the mouth and carcinoma of the testis. *Radiology* 67(Oct):484–497, 1956.

Michael, M., Jr. Epidemiology of sarcoidosis (Editorial). *Ann. Intern. Med.* 45(July):151–155, 1956.

Myers, J.A., Boynton, R.E., Kernan, P., Cowan, D., Jablon, S. Sensitivity to fungal antigens among students at the University of Minnesota. *Am. Rev. Tuberc.* 73(May):620–636, 1956.

Smetana, H.F., Cohen, B.M. Mortality in relation to histologic type in Hodgkin's disease. *Blood* 11(May):211–224, 1956.

VA Multiple Sclerosis Study Group. Isoniazid in the treatment of multiple sclerosis: Report on VA Cooperative Study. *Trans. Am. Neurol. Assoc.* 128–131, 1956.

1957

Beebe, G.W. Statistics and Clinical Investigation. Medical Bulletin (MB-2). Department of Medicine and Surgery, Veterans Administration, Washington, D.C., December 1957.

Myers, J.A., Boynton, R.E., Kernan, P., Cowan, D., Jablon, S. Sensitivity to tuberculin among students at the University of Minnesota. *Am. Rev. Tuberc.* 75(Mar.):442–460, 1957.

Palmer, C.E., Jablon, S., Edwards, P.Q. Tuberculosis morbidity of young men in relation to tuberculin sensitivity and body build. *Am. Rev. Tuberc.* 76(Oct.): 517–539, 1957.

VA Multiple Sclerosis Study Group. Isoniazid in the treatment of multiple sclerosis. *JAMA* 163(Jan.):168–172, 1957.

Woodhall, B., Beebe, G.W. (eds.) *Peripheral Nerve Regeneration: A Follow-up Study of 3,656 World War II Injuries.* VA Medical Monograph. Washington, D.C.: U.S. Government Printing Office, 1957.

Woodhall, B., Jablon, S. Prospects for further increase in average longevity. *Geriatrics* 12(Oct.):586–591, 1957.

1958

Michael, M., Jr. Sarcoidosis: Disease or syndrome. *Am. J. Med. Sci.* 235(Feb.): 148–153, 1958.

1959

Funkhouser, J.B., Nagler, B. The electroencephalogram of multiple sclerosis: A preliminary report. *Dis. Nerv. Syst.* 20(Jan.):41–44, 1959.

Walker, A.E., Jablon, S. A follow-up of head-injured men of World War II. *J. Neurosurg.* 16(Nov.):600–610, 1959.

1960

Beebe, G.W. Lung cancer in World War I veterans: Possible relation to mustard-gas injury and 1918 influenza epidemic. *J. Natl. Cancer Inst.* 25(Dec.):1231–1251, 1960.

Jenkins, R.L. The psychopathic or antisocial personality. *J. Nerv. Ment. Dis.* 131(Oct.):318–334, 1960.

Rubini, M.E., Jablon, S., McDowell, M.E. Renal residuals of acute epidemic hemorrhagic fever. *Arch. Intern. Med.* 106(Sept.):378–387, 1960.

Teuber, H.L., Battersby, W.S., Bender, M.B. *Visual Field Defects After Penetrating Missile Wounds of the Brain.* Cambridge, Mass: Harvard University Press, 1960.

1961

Elsom, K.A., Beebe, G.W., Sayen, J.J., Scheie, H.G., Gammon, G.D., Wood, F.C. Scrub typhus: A follow-up study. *Ann. Intern. Med.* 55(Nov.):784–795, 1961.

Heyman, A., Nefzger, M.D., Estes, H.E., Jr. Serum cholesterol level in cerebral infarction. *Arch. Neurol.* 5(Sept.):264–268, 1961.

Jablon, S. Characteristics of a Clinical Trial. In F.M. Forster (ed.) *Evaluation of Drug Therapy.* Madison: University of Wisconsin Press, 1961.

Kurtzke, J.F. On the evaluation of disability in multiple sclerosis. *Neurology* 11(Aug.):686–694, 1961.

Marshall, C., Walker, A.E. The value of electroencephalography in the prognostication and prognosis of post-traumatic epilepsy. *Epilepsia* 2:138–142, 1961.

VA Adjuvant Cancer Chemotherapy Cooperative Group. Status of adjuvant cancer chemotherapy: A preliminary report of cooperative studies in the Veterans Administration. *Arch. Surg.* 82(Mar.):466–473, 1961.

VA Cooperative Study of Atherosclerosis Group, Neurology Section. An evaluation of anticoagulant therapy in the treatment of cerebrovascular disease. *Neurology* 11(Apr.):132–138, 1961.

Walker, A.E., Jablon, S. *A Follow-up Study of Head Wounds in World War II.* VA Medical Monograph. Washington, D.C.: U.S. Government Printing Office, 1961.

1962

Bayani-Sioson, P.S., Louch, J., Sutton, H.E., Neel, J.V., Horne, S.L., Gershowitz, H. Quantitative studies on the haptoglobin of apparently healthy adult male twins. *Am. J. Hum. Genet.* 14(June):210–219, 1962.

Caveness, W.F., Walker, A.E., Ascroft, P.B. Incidence of post-traumatic epilepsy in Korean veterans as compared with those from World War I and World War II. *J. Neurosurg.* 19(Feb.):122–129, 1962.

Cohen, B.M., Neel, J.V., Gershowitz, H. Accuracy of World War II blood typing (Letter to the Editor). *Am. J. Hum. Genet.* 14(June):238–239, 1962.

DeBakey, M.E., Beebe, G.W. Medical follow-up studies on veterans. *JAMA* 182(Dec.):1103–1109, 1962.

Grossberg, S., Heyman, A., Keehn, R.J. Neurologic sequelae of Japanese encephalitis. *Trans. Am. Neurol. Assoc.* 87:114–117, 1962.

Hughes, F.A., Higgins, G. Veterans Administration Surgical Adjuvant Lung Cancer Chemotherapy Study: Present status. *J. Thorac. Cardiovasc. Surg.* 44(Sept.):295–308, 1962.

VA Adjuvant Study Group. Evaluation of chemotherapeutic agents as adjuvants to surgery in twenty-two Veterans Administration hospitals: Experimental design. *Cancer Chemother. Rep.* 20(July), 1962.

VA Adjuvant Study Group. The use of 5-fluoro-2'-deoxyuridine as a surgical adjuvant in carcinoma of the stomach and colon-rectum. *Cancer Chemother. Rep.* 24(Nov.):35–38, 1962.

Walker, A.E. Post-traumatic epilepsy. *World Neurol.* 3:185–194, 1962.

1963

Acheson, E.D., Nefzger, M.D. Ulcerative colitis in the United States Army in 1944. Epidemiology: Comparisons between cases and controls. *Gastroenterology* 44(Jan.):7–19 1963.

DeBakey, M.E., Cohen, B.M. *Buerger's Disease. A Follow-up Study of World War II Army Cases.* Springfield, Ill.: Charles C. Thomas, 1963.

Nagler, B., Beebe, G.W., Kurtzke, J.F., Auth, T.L., Kurland, L.T., Nefzger, M.D. Studies on the natural history of multiple sclerosis: objectives, designs, and methods. *Trans. Am. Neurol. Assoc.* 88:231–232, 1963.

Nefzger, M.D., Acheson, E.D. Ulcerative colitis in the United States Army in 1944. *Gut* 4:183–192, 1963.

Nefzger, M.D., Chalmers, T.C. The treatment of acute infectious hepatitis. *Am. J. Med.* 35(Sept.):299–309, 1963.

1964

Ad Hoc Committee of the Committee on Trauma, National Academy of Sciences–National Research Council, Division of Medical Sciences: Postoperative wound infections: The influence of ultraviolet irradiation of the operating room and of various other factors. *Ann. Surg.* 160(2, Suppl.), 1964.

Beebe, G.W., Simon, A.H., Vivona, S. Follow-up study on Army personnel who received adjuvant influenza virus vaccine 1951–1953. *Am. J. Med. Sci.* 247(Apr.):385–405, 1964.

Cohen, B.M., Smetana, H.F., Miller, R.W. Hodgkin's disease: Long survival in a study of 388 World War II Army cases. *Cancer* 17(July):856–866, 1964.

Dwight, R.W. Adjuvant chemotherapy in cancer of the large bowel. An interim report of the Veterans Administration Surgical Adjuvant Cancer Chemotherapy Study. *Am. J. Surg.* 107(Apr.):609–613, 1964.

Higgins, G.A., Flynn, T., Gillespie, J. Effect of splenectomy on tolerance to thiotepa. *Arch. Surg.* 88(Apr.):627–632, 1964.

VA Multiple Sclerosis Study Group. A five-year follow-up on multiple sclerosis. *Arch. Neurol.* 11(Dec.):583–592, 1964.

1965

Cleary, S.F., Pasternack, B.S., Beebe, G.W. Cataract incidence in radar workers. *Arch. Environ. Health* 11(Aug.):179–182, 1965.

Follow-up Agency. Federal agency probes health, medical history of ex-GI twins. *JAMA* 191(Mar.), 1965.

Schumacher, G.A., Beebe, G., Kibler, R.F., Kurland, L.T., Kurtzke, J.F., McDowell, F., Nagler, B., Sibley, W.A., Tourtellotte, W.W., Willmon, T.L. Problems of experimental trials of therapy in multiple sclerosis: Report by the Panel on the Evaluation of Experimental Trials of Therapy in Multiple Sclerosis. *Ann. NY Acad. Sci.* 122(Mar.):552–568, 1965.

VA Cooperative Surgical Adjuvant Study Group. Use of thio-tepa as an adjuvant to the surgical management of carcinoma of the stomach. *Am. Soc. Inc.* 18(3), 1965.

VA Surgical Adjuvant Cancer Chemotherapy Group. Adjuvant use of $HN_2(NSC-762)_1$ and thiotepa $(NSC-6396)_2$: Progress report. *Cancer Chemother. Rep.* 44(Feb.), 1965.

1966

Beebe, G.W., Rosen, D.I. The potential of the veteran population for epidemiologic studies on parkinsonism. *J. Neurosurg.* 24(Part 2, Jan.):144–148, 1966.

Bland, E.F., Beebe, G.W. Missiles in the heart: A twenty-year follow-up report of World War II cases. *N. Engl. J. Med.* 274(May):1039–1046, 1966.

Hughes, F., Higgins, G.A., Beebe, G.W. Present status of surgical adjuvant lung-cancer chemotherapy. *JAMA* 196(Apr.):343–344, 1966.

Kurland, L.T., Beebe, G.W., Kurtzke, J.F., Nagler, B., Auth, T.L., Lessell, S., Nefzger, M.D. Studies on the natural history of multiple sclerosis. 2: The progression of optic neuritis to multiple sclerosis. *Acta Neurol. Scand.* 42(Suppl. 19, Jan.):157–176, 1966.

Kurtzke, J.F. The distribution of multiple sclerosis and other diseases. *Acta Neurol. Scand.* 42:221–243, 1966.

Kurtzke, J.F., Beebe, G.W., Nagler, B., Auth, T.L., Kurland, L.T., Nefzger, M.D. Studies on the natural history of multiple sclerosis: The onset bout. *Trans. Am. Neurol. Assoc.* 91:278–280, 1966.

Nagler, B., Beebe, G.W., Kurtzke, J.F., Kurland, L.T., Auth, T.L., Nefzger, M.D. Studies on the natural history of multiple sclerosis. 1: Design and diagnosis. *Acta Neurol. Scand.* 42(Suppl. 19, Jan.):141–156, 1966.

1967

Beebe, G.W., Kurtzke, J.F., Kurland, L.T., Auth, T.L., Nagler, B. Studies on the natural history of multiple sclerosis. 3: Epidemiologic analysis of the Army experience in World War II. *Neurology* 17(Jan.):1–17, 1967.

Higgins, G.A., Beebe, G.W. Bronchogenic carcinoma: Factors in survival. *Arch. Surg.* 94(Apr.):539–549, 1967.

Jablon, S., Neel, J.V., Gershowitz, H., Atkinson, G.F. The NAS–NRC Twin Panel: Methods of construction of the panel: Zygosity diagnosis and proposed use. *Am. J. Hum. Genet.* 19(Mar.):133–161, 1967.

Nefzger, M.D., Heyman, A., LeBauer, J., Friedberg, S., Lewis, J. Serum cholesterol levels in myocardial and cerebral infarction caused by atherosclerosis. *J. Chronic Dis.* 20(Aug.):593–602, 1967.

1968

Higgins, G.A. Preoperative irradiation for lung carcinoma: The VA National Study. In B.F. Rush, Jr. and R.H. Greenlaw (eds.) *Cancer Therapy by Integrated Radiation and Operation.* Springfield, Ill.: Charles C. Thomas, 1968.

Higgins, G.A. Preoperative Irradiation for colo-rectal carcinoma: The VA National Study. In B.F. Rush, Jr. and R.H. Greenlaw (eds.) *Cancer Therapy by Integrated Radiation and Operation.* Springfield, Ill.: Charles C. Thomas, 1968.

Higgins, G.A., Dwight, R.W., Walsh, W.S., Humphrey, E.W. Preoperative radiation therapy as an adjuvant to surgery for carcinoma of the colon and rectum. *Am. J. Surg.* 115(Feb.):241–246, 1968.

Kurtzke, J.F., Beebe, G.W., Nagler, B., Auth, T.L., Kurland, L.T., Nefzger, M.D. Studies on natural history of multiple sclerosis. 4: Clinical features of the onset bout. *Acta Neurol. Scand.* 44:467–494, 1968.

Kurtzke, J.F., Beebe, G.W., Nagler, B., Kurland, L.T., Auth, T.L. Multiple sclerosis in United States Veterans: Preliminary observations. In M. Alter and J.F. Kurtzke (eds.) *The Epidemiology of Multiple Sclerosis.* Springfield, Ill.: Charles C. Thomas, 1968.

Nefzger, M.D., Quadfasel, F.A., Karl, V.C. A retrospective study of smoking in Parkinson's disease. *Am. J. Epidemiol.* 88(Sept.):149–158, 1968.

Warren, R., Kihn, R.B. A survey of lower extremity amputations for ischemia. *Surgery* 63(Jan.):107–120, 1968.

1969

Beebe, G.W., Simon, A.H. Ascertainment of mortality in the U.S. veteran population. *Am. J. Epidemiol.* 89(June):636–643, 1969.

Cederlof, R., Friberg, L., Hrubec, Z. Cardiovascular and respiratory symptoms in relation to tobacco smoking. A study on American twins. *Arch. Environ. Health* 18(June):934–940, 1969.

Dwight, R.W., Higgins, G.A., Keehn, R.J. Factors influencing survival following resection in cancer of the colon and rectum. *Am. J. Surg.* 117(Apr.):512–522, 1969.

Higgins, G.A., Humphrey, E.W., Hughes, F.A., Keehn, R.J. Cytoxan as an adjuvant to surgery for lung cancer. *J. Surg. Oncol.* 1:221–228, 1969.

Higgins, G.A., Lawton, R., Heilbrunn, A., Keehn, R.J. Prognostic factors in lung cancer: Surgical aspects. *Ann. Thorac. Surg.* 79(May):472–480, 1969.

Kurtzke, J.F. Some epidemiologic features compatible with an infectious origin for multiple sclerosis. In Pathogenesis and Etiology of Demyelinating Diseases. *Int. Arch. Allergy* 36(Suppl.):59–81, 1969.

Kurtzke, J.F., Auth, T.L., Beebe, G.W., Kurland, L.T., Nagler, B., Nefzger, M.D. Survival in multiple sclerosis. *Trans. Am. Neurol. Assoc.* 94:134–139, 1969.

Kurtzke, J.F., Beebe, G.W. Herpes zoster and multiple sclerosis (Letter to the Editor). *Br. Med. J.* 4(Nov.) 303, 1969.

Nefzger, M.D., Hrubec, Z., Chalmers, T.C. Venous thromboembolism and blood-group (Letter to the Editor). *Lancet* 1(Apr.):887, 1969.

Pollin, W., Allen, M.G., Hoffer, A., Stabenau, J.R., Hrubec, Z. Psychopathology in 15,909 pairs of veteran twins: Evidence for a genetic factor in the pathogenesis of schizophrenia and its relative absence in psychoneurosis. *Am. J. Psychiatry* 126(Nov.):597–610, 1969.

Serlin, O., Wolkoff, J.S., Amadeo, J.M., Keehn, R.J. Use of 5-fluorodeoxyuridine (FUDR) as an adjuvant to the surgical management of carcinoma of the stomach. *Cancer* 24(Aug.):223–228, 1969.

Zukel, W.J., Cohen, B.M., Mattingly, T.W., Hrubec, Z. Survival following first diagnosis of coronary heart disease. *Am. Heart J.* 78(Aug.):159–170, 1969.

1970

Allen, M.G., Pollin, W. Schizophrenia in twins and the diffuse ego boundary hypothesis. *Am. J. Psychiatry* 127(Oct.):437–442, 1970.

Beebe, G.W., Simon, A.H. Cirrhosis of the liver following viral hepatitis: a twenty-year mortality follow-up. *Am. J. Epidemiol.* 92(Nov.):279–286, 1970.

Feinleib, M., Havlik, R.J., Kwiterovich, P.O., Tillotson, J., Garrison, R.J. The National Heart Institute Twin Study. *Acta Genet. Med. Gemellol. (Roma)* 19:243–247, 1970.

Hoffer, A., Pollin, W. Schizophrenia in the NAS–NRC panel of 15,909 veteran twin pairs. *Arch. Gen. Psychiatry* 23(Nov.):469–477, 1970.

Kurtzke, J.F. Clinical manifestations of multiple sclerosis. In P.J. Vinken and G.W. Bruyn (eds.) *Handbook of Clinical Neurology*, Vol. 9: Multiple Sclerosis and Other Demyelinating Diseases. Amsterdam, North Holland Publishing Company, 1970.

Kurtzke, J.F. Neurologic impairment in multiple sclerosis and the disability status scale. *Acta Neurol. Scand.* 46:493–513, 1970.

Kurtzke, J.F., Beebe, G.W., Nagler, B., Nefzger, M.D., Auth, T.L., Kurland, L.T. Studies on the natural history of multiple sclerosis. V: Long-term survival in young men. *Arch. Neurol.* 22(Mar.):215–225, 1970.

Miller, R.W., Jablon, S. A search for late radiation effects among men who served as x-ray technologists in the U.S. Army during World War II. *Radiology* 96(Aug.):269–274, 1970.

Nashold, B.S., Jr. Summary report of a twenty year follow-up of Army men with lumbar disc disease. In E.S. Gurdjian and L.M. Thomas (eds.) *Neckache and Backache*. Proceedings of a Workshop Sponsored by the American Association of Neurological Surgeons in Cooperation with the National Institutes of Health. Springfield, Ill: Charles C. Thomas, 1970.

Nefzger, M.D. Follow-up studies of World War II and Korean War prisoners. 1: Study plan and mortality findings. *Am. J. Epidemiol.* 91(Feb.):123–138, 1970.

Reuling, F.H., Schwartz, J.T. Heritability of the effect of corticosteroids on intraocular pressure. *Acta Genet. Med. Gemellol. (Roma)* 19(Jan.–Apr.):264–267, 1970.

Roswit, B., Higgins, G.A., Keehn, R.J. A controlled study of preoperative irradiation in cancer of the sigmoid colon and rectum: Preliminary report. *Radiology* 97(Oct.):133–140, 1970.

Roswit, B., Higgins, G.A., Shields, T.W., Keehn, R.J. Preoperative radiation therapy for carcinoma of the lung: Report of a National VA Controlled Study. *Front. Radiat. Ther. Oncol.* 5:163–176, 1970.

Shields, T.W., Higgins, G.A., Lawton, R.L., Heilbrunn, A., Keehn, R.J. Preoperative x-ray therapy as an adjuvant in the treatment of bronchogenic carcinoma. *J. Thorac. Cardiovasc. Surg.* 59(Jan.):49–61, 1970.

Stabenau, J.R., Pollin, W., Allen, M.G. Twin studies in schizophrenia and neurosis. *Semin. Psychiatry* 2(Feb.) 65–74, 1970.

1971

Beebe, G.W. Linkage of wartime military and veterans records in cancer research. Pp. 364–376 in *Oncology, 1970: Environmental Causes, Epidemiology and Demography*. Cancer Education (Proceedings of the Tenth International Cancer Congress). Medical Publishers, 1971.

Burger, R.H., Smith, C. Hereditary and familial vesicoureteral reflux. *J. Urology.* 106(Dec.), 1971

Cederlof, R., Epstein, F.H., Friberg, L.T., Hrubec, Z., Radford, E.P. (eds.) Twin registries in the study of chronic disease. Report of an international symposium in San Juan, Puerto Rico, 1–4 December 1969. *Acta Med. Scand. Suppl.* 523, 1971.

Higgins, G.A., Dwight, R.W., Smith, J.D., Keehn, R.J. Fluorouracil as an adjuvant to surgery in carcinoma of the colon. *Arch. Surg.* 102(Apr.):339–343, 1971.

Hrubec, Z., Zukel, W.J. Socioeconomic differentials in prognosis following episodes of coronary heart disease. *J. Chronic Dis.* 23(May):881–889, 1971.

Nashold, B.S., Hrubec, Z. (eds.) *Lumbar Disc Disease: A Twenty Year Clinical Follow-up Study*. St. Louis: Mosby Company, 1971.

Nefzger, M.D. Mortality in World War II and Korean War prisoners. Pp. 36–52 in *Proceedings of the Second Medical and Juridical Conference of the German Documentation Center for Late Effects in Political and Military Prisoners*. Dusseldorf, March 20–22, 1969. Printed in German, 1971.

1972

Acheson, R.M., Nefzger, M.D., Heyman, A. Mortality from stroke among U.S. veterans in Georgia and five western states. V: Seventh and eighth revisions of the international classification of diseases as they relate to stroke. *Am. J. Epidemiol.* 96(Dec.):396–400, 1972.

Allen, M., Cohen, S., Pollin, W. Schizophrenia in veteran twins: A diagnostic review. *Am. J. Psychiatry* 128(Feb.):939–945, 1972.

Beebe, G.W., Simon, A.H., Vivona, S. Long-term mortality follow-up of Army recruits who received adjuvant influenza virus vaccine in 1951–1953. *Am. J. Epidemiol.* 95(Apr.):337–346, 1972.

Cohen, S.M., Allen, M.G., Pollin, W., Hrubec, Z. The relationship of schizo-affective psychosis to manic depressive psychosis and schizophrenia: Findings in 15,909 veteran twin pairs. *Arch. Gen. Psychiatry* 26(June):539–546, 1972.

Dwight, R.W., Higgins, G.A., Roswit, B., LeVeen, H.H., Keehn, R.J. Preoperative radiation and surgery for cancer of the sigmoid colon and rectum. *Am. J. Surg.* 123(Jan.):93–103, 1972.

Higgins, G.A., Jr. Use of chemotherapy as an adjuvant to surgery for bronchogenic carcinoma. *Cancer* 30(Nov.):1383–1387, 1972.

Higgins, G.A., Dwight, R.W. The role of preoperative irradiation in cancer of the rectum and rectosigmoid. *Surg. Clin. North Am.* 52(Aug.):847–858, 1972.

Hrubec, Z., Sutton, H.E. Smoking and health (Letter to the Editor). *Lancet* 2:932 (Oct.), 1972.

Kihn, R.B., Warren, R., Beebe, G.W. The "geriatric" amputee. *Ann. Surg.* 176(Sept.):305–314, 1972.

Kurtzke, J.F., Beebe, G.W., Nagler, B., Auth, T.L., Kurland, L.T., Nefzger, M.D. Studies on the natural history of multiple sclerosis. 6: Clinical and laboratory findings at first diagnosis. *Acta Neurol. Scand.* 48:19–46, 1972.

Jablon, S. Radiation cancers and A-bomb survivors (Letter to the Editor). *Lancet* 1(Feb.):375, 1972.

Lawton, R.L., Keehn, R.J. Bronchogenic cancer, sepsis, and survival. *J. Clin. Oncol.* 4 (May):466–469, 1972.

Nefzger, M.D., Mostofi, F.K. Survival after surgery for germinal malignancies of the testis. I: Rates of survival in tumor groups. *Cancer* 30(Nov.):1225–1232, 1972.

Nefzger, M.D., Mostofi, F.K. Survival after surgery for germinal malignancies of the testis. II: Effects of surgery and radiation. *Cancer* 30(Nov.):1233–1240, 1972.

Schwartz, J.T., Reuling, F.H., Feinleib, M., Garrison, R.J., Collie, D.J. Twin heritability study of the effect of corticosteroids on intraocular pressure. *J. Med. Genet.* 9(June):137–143, 1972.

Shields, T.W. Preoperative radiation therapy in the treatment of bronchial carcinoma. *Cancer* 30 (Nov.):1388–1394, 1972.

Shields, T.W., Higgins, G.A., Keehn, R.J. Factors influencing survival after resection for bronchial carcinoma. *J. Thorac. Cardiovasc. Surg.* 64 (Sept.):391–399, 1972.

VA Cooperative Study of Atherosclerosis Group, Neurology Section. Estrogenic therapy in men with ischemic cerebrovascular disease: Effect on recurrent cerbral infarction and survival. *Stroke* 3(July–Aug.):427–433, 1972.

Waters, T.D., Anderson, P.S., Jr., Beebe, G.W., Miller, R.W. Yellow fever vaccination, avian leukosis virus and cancer risk in man. *Science* 177(July):76–77, 1972.

1973

Acheson, R.M., Heyman, A., Nefzger, M.D. Mortality from stroke among U.S. veterans in Georgia and five western states. III: Hypertension and demographic characteristics. *J. Chronic Dis.* 26 (July):417–429, 1973.

Acheson, R.M., Nefzger, M.D., Heyman, A. Mortality from stroke among U.S. veterans in Georgia and five western states. II: Quality of death certification and clinical records. *J. Chronic Dis.* 26(July):405–415, 1973.

Dwight, R.W., Humphrey, E.W., Higgins, G.A., Keehn, R.J. FUDR as an adjuvant to surgery in cancer of the large bowel. *J. Surg. Oncol.* 5(May):243–249, 1973.

Heyman, A., Nefzger, M.D., Acheson, R.M. Mortality from stroke among U.S. veterans in Georgia and five western states. IV: Clinical observations. *J. Chronic Dis.* 26(July):431–446, 1973.

Heyman, A., Nefzger, M.D., Acheson, R.M., Diamond, E.L. Mortality of stroke among U.S. veterans in Georgia and five western states. VI: Criteria and guidelines for automated diagnosis of stroke from medical records. *Neurology* 23(Nov.):1174–1181, 1973.

Hrubec, Z. The effect of diagnostic ascertainment in twins on the assessment of the genetic factor in disease etiology. *Am. J. Hum. Genet.* 25(Jan.):15–28, 1973.

Hrubec, Z. Coffee drinking and ischaemic heart disease (Letter to the Editor). *Lancet* 1(Mar.):548, 1973.

Hrubec, Z., Cederlof, R., Friberg, L. Respiratory symptoms in twins: Effects of residence-associated air pollution, tobacco and alcohol use, and other factors. *Arch. Environ. Health* 27(Sept.):189–195, 1973.

Jablon, S. Cancer as a late effect of radiation. In Proceedings of the 39th Session, International Statistical Institute Meeting, Vienna, Austria. *Bull. Int. Stat. Inst.* 45:135–144, 1973.

Jablon, S. Comments on "The carcinogenic effects of low level radiation. A re-appraisal of epidemiologists methods and observations." *Health Phys.* 24 (Feb.):257–258, 1973.

Jablon, S. Late Mortality Effects of Radiation in Man. In *Health Physics in the Healing Arts.* Health Physics Society Seventh Midyear Topical Symposium. San Juan, Puerto Rico, December 1972. DHEW Publication No. (FDA) 73-8029 Washington, D.C., 1973.

Jablon, S. The Origin and Findings of the Atomic Bomb Casualty Commission. A Lecture. DHEW Publication No. (FDA) 73-8032, Washington, D.C., 1973.

Jablon, S. The origin and findings of the Atomic Bomb Casualty Commission. *Nucl. Safety* 14(Nov.–Dec.):651–659, 1973.

Kurtzke, J.F., Beebe, G.W., Nagler, B., Auth, T.L., Kurland, L.T., and Nefzger, M.D. Studies on the natural history of multiple sclerosis. 7: Correlates of clinical change in an early bout. *Acta Neurol. Scand.* 49:379–395, 1973.

Lawton, R.L. A case for interoperative radiation for the treatment of clinically operable, nonresectable bronchogenic carcinoma. *The Journal of Thoracic and Cardiovascular Surgery* 65(3):449–452, 1973

Matthews, M.J., Kanhauwa, S., Pickren, J., Robinette, D. Frequency of residual and metastatic tumor in patients undergoing curative surgical resection for lung cancer. *Cancer Chemother. Rep.* 4 (Mar.):63–67, 1973.

Miller, R.W., Beebe, G.W. Infectious mononucleosis and the empirical risk of cancer. *JNCI* 50 (Feb.):315–321, 1973.

Nefzger, M.D., Acheson, R.M., Heyman, A. Mortality from stroke among U.S. veterans in Georgia and five western states. I: Study plan and death rates. *J. Chronic Dis.* 26 (July):393–404, 1973.

Roswit, B., Higgins, G.A., Humphrey, E.W., Robinette, C.D. Preoperative irra-diation of operable adenocarcinoma of the rectum and rectosigmoid colon: Report of a randomized study. *Radiology* 108(Aug.):389–395, 1973.

Schwartz, J.T., Reuling, F.H., Feinleib, M., Garrison, R.J., Collie, D.J. Twin heritability study of corticosteroid response. *Trans. Am. Acad. Opthalmol. Otolaryngol.* 77(Mar.–Apr.):126–136, 1973.

Schwartz, J.T., Reuling, F.H., Feinleib, M., Garrison, R.J., Collie, D.J. Twin study on ocular pressure after topical dexamethasone. I: Frequency distribu-tion of pressure response. *Am. J. Opthalmol.* 76(July):126–136, 1973.

Schwartz, J.T., Reuling, F.H., Feinleib, M., Garrison, R.J., Collie, D.J. Twin study on ocular pressure following topically applied dexamethasone. II: In-heritance of variation in pressure response. *Arch. Ophthalmol.* 90(Oct.):281–286, 1973.

Shields, T.W., Robinette, C.D. Long term survivors after resection for bronchial carcinoma. *Surg. Gynecol. Obstet.* 136(May):759–762, 1973.

Smith, D.M., Nance, W.E., Kang, K.W., Christian, J.C., Jr. Genetic factors in determining bone mass. *J. Clin. Invest.* 52:2800–2808, 1973

Wyatt, R.J., Murphy, D.L., Belmaker, R., Cohen, S., Donnelly, C.H., Pollin, W. Reduced monoamine oxidase activity in platelets: A possible genetic marker for vulnerability to schizophrenia. *Science* 173(March):916–918, 1973.

1974

Bazaral, M., Orgel, H.A., Hamburger, R.N. Genetics of IgE and allergy: Serum IgE levels in twins. *J. Allergy Clin. Immunol.* 54(Nov.):288–304, 1974.

Bingle, G.J. The inheritance of electrocardiographic variables in man: A comparison of twin and half-sib models. Ph.d. thesis. Indiana University, 1974.

Feinleib, M. The analysis and interpretation of twin heritability studies. Pp. 49–59 in M. Goldberg (ed.) *Genetic and Metabolic Eye Disease.* Boston: Little, Brown & Co., 1974.

Hrubec, Z., Zukel, W.J. Epidemiology of coronary heart disease among young Army males of World War II. *Am. Heart J.* 87(June):722–730, 1974.

Keehn, R.J. Probability of death related to previous Army rank (Letter to the Editor). *Lancet* 2(July):170, 1974.

Keehn, R.J., Goldberg, I.D., Beebe, G.W. Twenty-four year mortality follow-up of Army veterans with disability separations for psychoneurosis in 1944. *Psychosom. Med.* 36(Jan.–Feb.):27–46, 1974.

King, R.J. The efficiency of human twins in studies of associations between plasma lipids and genetic markers. Ph.D. thesis. Indiana University, 1974.

Lynfield, Y.L. Skin diseases in twins. *Arch. Dermatol.* 110(Nov.):722–724, 1974.

Rahe, R.H., Rosenman, R.H., Borhani, N.O., Feinleib, M. Heritability and psychologic correlates of behavior pattern types A and B. (Abstract). *Am. J. Epidemiol.* 100:521–522, 1974.

Schwartz, J.T., Feinleib, M. Twin Heritability Study. Pp. 37–58 in M. Goldberg (ed.) *Genetic and Metabolic Eye Disease.* Boston: Little, Brown & Co., 1974.

Seltzer, C.C., Jablon, S. Effects of selection on mortality. *Am. J. Epidemiol.* 100(Nov.):367–372, 1974.

Shields, T.W. The fate of patients after incomplete resection of bronchial carcinoma. *Surg. Gynecol. Obstet.* 139(Oct.):569–572, 1974.

Shields, T.W., Robinette, C.D., Keehn, R.J. Bronchial carcinoma treated by adjuvant cancer chemotherapy. *Arch. Surg.* 109(Aug.):329–333, 1974.

1975

Beebe, G.W. Follow-up studies of World War II and Korean War prisoners. II: Morbidity, disability, and maladjustments. *Am. J. Epidemiol.* 101(May):400–422, 1975.

Bohning, D.E., Albert, R.E., Lippmann, M., Foster, W.M. Tracheobronchial particle deposition and clearance. *Arch. Environ. Health* 30(Sept.):457–462, 1975.

Cheung, S.W. Biochemical and Genetic Studies of Human High Density Plasma Lipoproteins. Ph.D. thesis, Indiana University, 1975.

Christian, J.C., Feinleib, M., Norton, J.A., Jr. Statistical analysis of genetic variance in twins. *Am. J. Hum. Genet.* 27:807, 1975.

Feinleib, M., Garrison, R., Borhani, N., Rosenman, R., Christian, J. Studies of Hypertension in Twins. In P. Oglesby (ed.) *Epidemiology and Control of Hypertension.* Second International Symposium on the Epidemiology of Hypertension, September 1974. Miami: Symposia Specialists, 1975.

Higgins, G.A., Conn, J.H., Jordan, P.H., Humphrey, E.W., Roswit, B., Keehn, R.J. Preoperative radiotherapy for colorectal cancer. *Ann. Surg.* 181(May): 624–631, 1975.

Higgins, G.A., Shields, T.W., Keehn, R.J. The solitary pulmonary nodule: Ten-year follow-up of Veterans Administration–Armed Forces Cooperative Study. *Arch. Surg.* 110(May):570–575, 1975.

Hrubec, Z., Allen, G. Methods and interpretation of twin concordance data (Letter to the Editor). *Am. J. Hum. Genet.* 27(Nov.):808–809, 1975.

Hrubec, Z., Nashold, B. Epidemiology of lumbar disc lesions in the military in World War II. *Am. J. Epidemiol.* 102(Nov.):366–376, 1975.

Jablon, S. Environmental factors in cancer induction: Appraisal of epidemiologic evidence. Leukemia, lymphoma, and radiation. Pp. 239–243 in *Proceedings of the Eleventh International Cancer Congress,* Vol. 3, *Cancer Epidemiology: Environmental Factors.* Amsterdam, 1975.

Jablon, S. The late effects of acute external exposure to ionzing radiation in man. Pp. 132–145 in O.F. Nygaard, H.I. Adler and W.K. Sinclair (eds.) *Radiation Research: Biomedical, Chemical and Physical Perspectives.* New York: Academic Press, 1975.

Jablon, S. Radiation. Pp. 151–165 in J.F. Fraumeni, Jr. (ed.) *Persons at High Risk of Cancer: An Approach to Cancer Etiology and Control.* New York: Academic Press, 1975.

McCune, S.A. Genetic studies of human aminoacyl transfer ribonucleic acid synthetases from erythrocytes and placentae of normal twins. Ph.D. thesis, Indiana University, 1975.

Norman, J.E., Jr. Lung cancer mortality in World War I veterans with mustard-gas injury: 1919–1965. *JNCI* 54(Feb.):311–317, 1975.

Paul, T.D. Analysis of the inheritance of normal human serum amino acid levels by the twin study method. M.S. thesis, Indiana University, 1975.

Reed, T., Sprague, F.R., Kang, K.W., Nance, W.E., Christian, J.C. Genetic analysis of dermatoglyphics patterns in twins. *Hum. Hered.* 25:263–275, 1975.

Roswit, B., Higgins, G.A., Keehn, R.J. Preoperative irradiation for carcinoma of the rectum and rectosigmoid colon: Report of a national VA randomized study. *Cancer* 35(June):1597–1602, 1975.

Seltzer, C.C., Jablon, S. Effects of selection on mortality (Letter to the Editor). *Am. J. Epidemiol.* 102(Sept.):263–264, 1975.

Shields, T.W., Yee, J., Conn, J.H., Robinette, C.D. Relationship of cell type and lymph node metastasis to survival after resection of bronchial carcinoma. *Ann. Thorac. Surg.* 20(Nov.):501–510, 1975.

Ziegler, D.K., Hassanein, R.S., Harris, D., Stewart, R. Headache in a non-clinic twin population. *Headache* 14(Jan.):213–218, 1975.

1976

Borhani, N.O., Feinleib, M., Garrison, R.J., Christian, J.C., Rosenman, R.H. Genetic variance in blood pressure. *Acta Genet. Med. Gemellol. (Roma)* 25:137–144, 1976.

Christian, J.C., Feinleib, M., Hulley, S.B., Castelli, W.P., Fabsitz, R.R., Garrison, R.J., Borhani, N.O., Rosenman, R.H., Wagner, J. Genetics of plasma cholesterol and triglycerides: A study of adult male twins. *Acta Genet. Med. Gemellol. (Roma)* 25:145–149, 1976.

Feinleib, M. Twin Studies. Pp. 59–82 in M. Feinleib and B.M. Rifkind (eds.) *Report from the NHLI Task Force on Genetic Factors in Atherosclerotic Disease.* Publication No. (NIH) 76-922. Washington, D.C.: U.S. Dept. of Health, Education & Welfare, 1976.

Feinleib, M., Christian, J.C., Borhani, N.O., Rosenman, R., Garrison, R.J., Wagner, J., Kannel, W.B., Hrubec, Z., Schwartz, J.T. The National Heart and Lung Institute Twin Study of Cardiovascular Disease Risk Factors: Organization and methodology. *Acta Genet. Med. Gemellol. (Roma)* 25:125–128, 1976.

Higgins, G.A., Jr., Humphrey, E., Juler, G.L., LeVeen, H.H., McCaughan, J., Keehn, R.J. Adjuvant chemotherapy in the surgical treatment of large bowel cancer. *Cancer* 38(Oct.):1461–1467, 1976.

Higgins, G.A., Jr., Serlin, O., Amadeo, J.H., McElhinney, J.L., Keehn, R.J. Gastric cancer: Factors in survival. *Chir. Gastroenterol. (Surg. Gastroenterol)* 10:393–398, 1976.

Horn, J.M., Plomin, R., Rosenman, R. Heritability of personality traits in adult male twins. *Behav. Genet.* 6:17–30, 1976.

Hrubec, Z., Cederlof, R., Friberg, L. Background of angina pectoris: Social and environmental factors in relation to smoking. *Am. J. Epidemiol.* 103(Jan.):16–29, 1976.

Huntzinger, R.S. The inheritance of retinal blood vessel patterns in man: A twin study. Ph.D. thesis, Indiana University, 1976.

Rosenman, R.H., Rahe, R.H., Borhani, N.O., Feinleib, M. Heritability of personality and behavior pattern. *Acta Genet. Med. Gemellol. (Roma)* 25:221–224, 1976.

Sprague, F.R. Dermatoglyphic patterns of fingers, palms and soles: Analysis of genetic variance in twins and use in zygosity determination. M.S. thesis, Indiana University, 1976.

Taubman, P. The determinants of earnings: Genetics, family and other environments: A study of white male twins. *Am. Economic Rev.* 66(Dec.):858–870, 1976.

Taubman, P. Earnings, education, genetics, and environment. *J. Hum. Resour.* 11(fall):447–461, 1976.

1977

Behrman, J., Taubman, P., Wales, T. Controlling for and measuring the effects of genetics and family environment in equations for schooling and labor market success. In P. Taubman (ed.) *Kinometrics: Determinants of Socioeconomic Success Within and Between Families.* New York: North-Holland Publishing Company, 1977.

Boklage, C.E. Schizophrenia, brain asymmetry development, and twinning: Cellular relationship with etiological and possibly prognostic implications. *Biol. Psychiatry* 12(1):19–35, 1977.

Feinleib, M., Garrison, R.J., Fabsitz, R., Christian, J.C., Hrubec, Z., Borhani, N.O., Kannel, W.B., Rosenman, R., Schwartz, J.T., Wagner, J.O. The NHLBI Twin Study of Cardiovascular Disease Risk Factors: Methodology and summary of results. *Am. J. Epidemiol.* 106(Oct.):284–295, 1977.

Havlik, R.J., Garrison, R.J., Fabsitz, R.R., Feinleib, M. Genetic variability of clinical chemical values. *Clin. Chem.* 23:659–662, 1977.

Kurtzke, J.F., Beebe, G.W., Nagler, B., Kurland, L.T., Auth, T.L. Studies on the natural history of multiple sclerosis. 8: Early prognostic features of the later course of the illness. *J. Chronic Dis.* 30(Dec.):819–830, 1977.

Reed, T., Norton, J.A., Jr., Christian, J.C. Sources of information for discriminating MZ and DZ twins by dermatoglyphic patterns. *Acta Genet. Med. (Roma)* 26:83–86, 1977.

Robinette, C.D., Fraumeni, J.F., Jr. Splenectomy and subsequent mortality in veterans of the 1939–45 War. *Lancet* 2(July):127–129, 1977.

Robinette, C.D., Silverman, C. Causes of death following occupational exposure to microwave radiation (RADAR) 1950–1974. Pp. 338–344 in D.G. Hazzard (ed.) *Symposium on Biological Effects and Measurements of Radio Frequency/Microwaves.* DHEW Publication No. (FDA) 77-8026. Washington, D.C.: Department of Health, Education, and Welfare, July 1977.

Seltzer, C.C., Jablon, S. Army rank and subsequent mortality by cause: 23-year follow-up. *Am. J. Epidemiol.* 105(June):559–566, 1977.

Serlin, O., Keehn, R.J., Higgins, G.A., Jr., Harrower, H.W., Mendeloff, G.L. Factors related to survival following resection for gastric carcinoma: Analysis of 903 cases. *Cancer* 40(Sept.):1318–1329, 1977.

Shields, T.W., Humphrey, E.W., Keehn, R.J. Adjuvant cancer chemotherapy after resection of carcinoma of the lung. *Cancer* 40(Nov.):2057–2062, 1977.

Shields, T.W., Keehn, R.J. Postresection stage grouping in carcinoma of the lung. *Surg. Gynecol. Obstet.* 145(Nov.):725–728, 1977.

1978

Asano, M., Norman, J.E., Kato, H., Yagawa, K. Autopsy studies of Hashimoto's thyroiditis in Hiroshima and Nagasaki (1954–1974), Relation to atomic bomb radiation. *J. Radiat. Res.* 19:306–318, 1978.

Bobowick, A.R., Kurtzke, J.F., Brody, J.A., Hrubec, Z., Gillespie, M. Twin study of multiple sclerosis: An epidemiologic inquiry. *Neurology* 28(Oct.):978–987, 1978.

Fabsitz, R.R., Feinleib M., Garrison, R.J. An evaluation of the intrapair relationship for personal attributes in the NHLBI twin study. Pp. 71–80 in W.E. Nance, G. Allen, and P. Parisi (eds.) *Twin Research. Part B. Biology and Epidemiology.* New York: Alan R. Liss, 1978.

Fabsitz, R.R., Garrison, R.J., Feinleib, M., Hjortland, M. A twin analysis of dietary intake: Evidence for a need to control for possible environmental differences in MZ and DZ Twins. *Behav. Genet.* 8(Jan.):15–25, 1978.

Feinleib, M., Ware, J.H., Garrison, R.J., Borhani, N.O., Christian, J.C., Rosenman, R. An analysis of variance for major coronary heart disease risk factors in twins and their brothers. Pp. 13–19 in W.E. Nance (ed.) *Twin Research.* Proceedings of the Second International Congress on Twin Studies, August 29–September 1, 1977, Washington, D.C., Part C. *Clinical Studies, Progress in Clinical and Biological Research*, Volume 24C. New York: Alan R. Liss, 1978.

Garrison, R.J., Demets, D.L., Fabsitz, R.R., Feinleib, M. A likelihood ratio test for unequal shared environmental variance in twin studies. Pp. 253–259 in W.E. Nance, G. Allen, P. Parisi, (eds.) *Twin Research. Part A. Psychology and Methodology.* New York, Alan R. Liss, Inc., 1978.

Higgins, G.A., Jr., Humphrey, E.W., Amadeo, J.H., Juler, G.L. Preoperative radiotherapy for colorectal cancer. Pp. 167–170 in A. Gerard (ed.) *Gastrointestinal Tumors: A Clinical and Experimental Approach.* Proceedings of an International Symposium sponsored by the European Organization for Research and Treatment of Cancer, Brussels, April 14–15, 1977. Brussels, Belgium: Institut Jules Bordet, 1978.

Higgins, G.A., Jr., Lee, L.E., Jr., Dwight, R.W., Keehn, R.J. The case for adjuvant 5-fluorouracil in colorectal cancer. *Cancer Clin. Trials* 1(spring)35–41, 1978.

Higgins, G.A., Jr., LeVeen, H.H., McCaughan, J., McElhinney, J. Adjuvant 5-fluorouracil in large bowel cancer. Pp. 171–175 in A. Gerard (ed.) *Gastrointestinal Tumors: A Clinical and Experimental Approach.* Proceedings of an International Symposium sponsored by the European Organization for

Research and Treatment of Cancer, Brussels, April 14–15, 1977, Brussels: Institut Jules Bordet, 1978.

Hrubec, Z., Neel, J.V. The National Academy of Sciences–National Research Council Twin Registry: Ten years of operation. Pp. 153–172 in W.E. Nance (ed.) *Twin Research*. Proceedings of the Second International Congress on Twin Studies, August 29–September 1, 1977, Washington, D.C., Part B. *Biology and Epidemiology, Progress in Clinical and Biological Research*, Volume 24B. New York: Alan R. Liss, 1978.

Jablon, S., Miller, R.W. Army technologists: 29-year follow-up for cause of death. *Radiology* 126 (Mar.):677–679, 1978.

Keehn, R.J. Military rank at separation and mortality. *Armed Forces and Society* 4(Feb.):283–292, 1978.

King, R.J., Garrison, R.J., Feinleib, M., Christian, J.C. Studies of association between genetic markers and plasma lipids in twins. Pp. 165–170 in W.E. Nance, G. Allen, and P. Parisi (eds.) *Twin Research*. Part C. *Clinical Studies*. New York: Alan R. Liss, 1978.

Land, C.E., Norman, J.E. Pp. 29–47 in *Latent Periods of Radiogenic Cancers Occurring Among Japanese A-Bomb Survivors*. Vienna: International Atomic Energy Agency, 1978.

Lieberman, J., Borhani, N.O., Feinleib, M. Twinning as heterozygous advantage for alpha-antitrypsin deficiency. Pp. 45–54 in W.E. Nance, G. Allen, and P. Parisi (eds.) *Twin Research*. Part B. *Biology and Epidemiology*. New York: Alan R. Liss, 1978.

Miller, L.H., McGinniss, M.H., Holland, P.V., Sigmon, P. The Duffy blood group phenotype in American blacks infected with plasmodium vivax in Vietnam. *Am. J. Trop. Med. Hyg.* 27:1069–1072, 1978.

Paul, T.D., Brandt, I.K., Christian, J.C., Jackson, C.E., Nance, C.S., Nance, W.E. Analysis of serum amino-acid levels by the twin study method and comparison with family studies. *Progress Clin. Biol. Res.* 24C:157–163, 1978.

Rahe, R.H., Hervig, L., Rosenman, R.H. Heritability of Type A behavior. *Psychosom. Med.* 40(Oct.):478–486, 1978.

Reed, T., Norton, J.A., Jr., Christian, J.C. Fingerprint pattern factors. *Human Hered.* 28:351–360, 1978.

Robinette, C.D., Fraumeni, J.F., Jr. Asthma and subsequent mortality in World War II veterans. *J. Chronic Dis.* 31(June):619–624, 1978.

Shields, T.W., Humphrey, E.W., Higgins, G.A., Jr., Keehn, R.J. Long-term survivors after resection of lung carcinoma. *J. Thorac. Cardiovasc. Surg.* 76(Oct.): 439–445, 1978.

Taubman, P. What we learn from estimating the genetic contribution to inequality in earnings: Reply. *Am. Econ. Rev.* 68(Dec.):970–976, 1978.

1979

Allen, G., Hrubec, Z. Twin concordance: A more general model. *Acta Genet. Med. Gemellol.* 28:3–13, 1979.

Boice, D., Jr., Land, C.E., Shore, R.E., Norman, J.E., Tokunaga, M. Risk of breast cancer following low-dose radiation exposure. *Radiology* 131(3): 589–597, 1979.

Cook, S.D., Dowling, P.C., Norman, J., Jablon, S. Multiple sclerosis and canine distemper in Iceland (Letter to the Editor). *Lancet* 1(Feb.):380–381, 1979.

Havlik, R.J., Garrison, R.J., Katz, S.H., Ellison, R.C., Feinleib, M., Myrianthopoulos N.C. Detection of genetic variance in blood pressure of seven-year-old twins. *Am. J. Epidemiol.* 109:512–516, 1979.

Higgins, G.A. Adjuvant Radiation Therapy in Colon Cancer. Pp. 1–24 in *International Advances in Surgical Oncology*, Vol. 2. New York: Alan R. Liss, Inc., 1979.

Higgins, G.A., Jr., Shields, T.W. Experience of the Veterans Administration Surgical Adjuvant Group. Pp. 433–442 in F. Muggia and M. Rozencweig (eds.) *Lung Cancer: Progress in Therapeutic Research.* New York: Raven Press, 1979.

Hrubec, Z., Ryder, R.A. Report to the Veterans Administration Department of Medicine and Surgery on service-connected traumatic limb amputations and subsequent mortality from cardiovascular disease and other causes of death. *Bull. Prosthet. Res.* 16(fall):29–53, 1979.

Humphrey, E.W., Keehn, R.J., Higgins, G.A., Jr., Shields, T.W. The long term survival of patients with visceral cancer. *Surg. Gynecol. Obstet.* 149(Sept.): 385–394, 1979.

Hutchison, G.B., MacMahon, B., Jablon, S., Land, C.E. Review of report by Mancuso, Stewart and Kneale of radiation exposure of Hanford workers. *Health Phys.* 37(Aug.):207–220, 1979.

Jablon, S. Comments on "Leukemia risk from neutrons" by Rossi, H.H. and Mays, C.W. (Letter to the Editor). *Health Phys.* 36(Feb.):205–206, 1979.

Kurtzke, J.F., Beebe, G.W., Norman, J.E., Jr. Epidemiology of multiple sclerosis in U.S. veterans 1: Race, sex, and geographic distribution. *Neurology* 29(Sept.):1228–1235, 1979.

Reed, T., Christian, J.C. Quantitative twin analysis of radial and ulnar ridge counts and ridge count diversity. *Acta. Genet. Med. Gemellol.* 28:165–168, 1979.

Reed, T., Norton, J.A., Jr., Christian, J.C. Dermatoglyphic pattern factors. In W.Wertelecki and C.C. Plato (eds.) Dermatoglyphics—50 Years Later. *Birth Defects Orig. Art Ser.* XV(6):85–93, 1979.

Reed, T. Young, R.S. Genetic analysis of multivariate fingertip dermatoglyphic factors and comparison with corresponding individual variables. *Ann. Hum. Biol.* 6:357–362, 1979.

Robinette, C.D., Hrubec, Z., Fraumeni, J.F., Jr. Chronic alcoholism and subsequent mortality in World War II veterans. *Am. J. Epidemiol.* 109(June):687–700, 1979.

Tokunaga, M., Norman, J.E., Asano, M., Tokuoka, S., Ezaki, H., Nishimori, I., Tsuji, Y. Malignant breast tumors among atomic bomb survivors, Hiroshima and Nagasaki, 1950–1974. *JNCI* 62(6):1347–1359, 1979.

Tolley, H.D., Norman, J.E. Time on trial estimates with bivariate risks. *Biometrika.* 66(2):285–291, 1979.

1980

Anderson, R.E., Hill, R.B., Hrubec, Z. Prospects for pathology studies in the NAS–NRC Twin Registry. *Hum. Pathol.* 11(Sept.):403, 1980.

Boice, J.D., Greene, M.H., Keehn, R.J., Higgins, G.A., Fraumeni, J.F., Jr. Late effects of low dose adjuvant chemotherapy in colorectal cancer. *JNCI* 64(Mar.):501–511, 1980.

Fabsitz, R., Feinleib, M., Hrubec, Z. Weight changes in adult twins. *Acta Genet. Med. Gemellol.* 29:273–279, 1980.

Foch, T.T., McClearn, G.E. Genetics, body weight, and obesity. Pp. 48–71 in A.J. Stunkard (ed.) *Obesity.* Philadelphia, Saunders, 1980.

Havlik, R.J., Garrison, R.J., Fabsitz, R., Feinleib, M. Variability of heart rate, P-R, QRS, and Q-T durations in twins. *J. Electrocardiol.* 13:45–48, 1980.

Hrubec, Z. The Data. In J.R. Behrman, Z. Hrubec, P. Taubman, and T.J. Wales (eds.) *Socioeconomic Success: A Study of the Effects of Genetic Endowments, Family Environment, and Schooling.* Amsterdam: North-Holland Publishing Company, 1980.

Hrubec, Z., Omenn, G.S. Evidence of genetic predisposition to alcoholic cirrhosis and psychosis: Twin concordances for alcoholism and its biologic end points by zygosity among male veterans (Abstract of paper presented at Thirty-first Annual Meeting, American Society of Human Genetics, New York, September 1980). *Am. J. Hum. Genet.* 32(Nov.):112A, 1980.

Hrubec, Z., Ryder, R.A. Traumatic limb amputations and subsequent mortality from cardiovascular disease and other causes. *J. Chronic Dis.* 33:239–250, 1980.

Hubert, H.B., Fabsitz, R.R., Feinleib, M., Brown, K.S. Olfactory sensitivity in humans: Genetic versus environmental control. *Science* 208(May):607–609, 1980.

Jablon, S., Bailar, J.C., III. The contribution of ionizing radiation to cancer mortality in the United States. *Prev. Med.* 9(Mar.):219–226, 1980.

Keehn, R.J. Follow-up Studies of World War II and Korean conflict prisoners. III: Mortality to 1 January 1976. *Am. J. Epidemiol.* 111(Feb.):194–211, 1980.

Kurtzke, J.F., Beebe, G.W. Epidemiology of amyotrophic lateral sclerosis 1: A case-control comparison based on ALS deaths. *Neurology* 30(May):453–462, 1980.

Robinette, C.D., Silverman, C., Jablon, S. Effects upon health of occupational exposure to microwave radiation (RADAR). *Am. J. Epidemiol.* 112(July):39–53, 1980.

Shields, T.W., Humphrey, E.W., Matthews, M., Eastridge, C.E., Keehn, R.J. Pathological stage grouping of patients with resected carcinoma of the lung. *J. Thorac. Cardiovasc. Surg.* 80(Sept.):400–405, 1980.

1981

Frey, C., Twomey, P., Keehn, R., Elliott, D., Higgins, G. Randomized study of 5-FU and CCNU in pancreatic cancer: Report of the Veterans Administration Surgical Adjuvant Cancer Chemotherapy Study Group. *Cancer* 47(Jan.):27–31, 1981.

Higgins, G.A., Donaldson, R.C., Humphrey, E.W., Rogers, L.S., Shields, T.W. Adjuvant therapy for large bowel cancer: Update of Veterans Administration Surgical Oncology Group Trials. *Surg. Clin. North Am.* 61(Dec.):1311–1320, 1981.

Higgins, G.A., Humphrey, E.W., Juler, G.L., Roswit, B., Keehn, R.J. Adjuvant therapy for rectal cancer: Update of Veterans Administration Surgical Oncology Group Trials. Pp. 62–67 in A. Gerard (ed.) *Progress and Perspectives in the Treatment of Gastrointestinal Tumors.* New York: Pergamon Press, 1981.

Horn, J.M., Matthews, K., Rosenman, R. Blood groups, physical appearance and personality similarity in adult dizygotic twins. In *Twin Research. 3: Intelligence, Personality and Development.* New York: Alan R. Liss, 1981.

Hrubec, Z. Methodologic problems in matched-pair studies using twins. Pp. 1–7 in L. Gedda, P. Parisi, and W.E. Nance (eds.) *Twin Research. 3: Part C: Epidemiological and Clinical Studies: Progress in Clinical and Biological Research.* Volume 69C. New York: Alan R. Liss, 1981.

Hrubec, Z., Neel, J.V. Familial factors in early deaths: Twins followed 30 years to ages 51–61 in 1978. *Hum. Genet.* 59:39–46, 1981.

Hrubec, Z., Omenn, G.S. Evidence of genetic predisposition to alcoholic cirrhosis and psychosis: Twin concordances for alcoholism and its biological end points by zygosity among male veterans alcoholism. *Clinical and Experimental Research* 5(spring):207–215, 1981.

Jablon, S. Radiation estimates (Letter to the Editor). *Science* 213(July):6, 1981.

Keehn, R.J., Higgins, G.A., Jr. Chemotherapy for gastric cancer (Letter to the Editor). *Lancet* 1(Feb.):323, 1981.

Norman, J.E., Jr., Robinette, C.D., Fraumeni, J.F., Jr. The mortality experience of Army World War II chemical processing companies. Pp. 312–322 in *Proceedings of the Eleventh Conference on Environmental Toxicology,* November 18–20, 1980, Dayton, Ohio. USAF Publication No. AFAMRL-TR-80-125, 1981,

Norman, J.E., Jr., Robinette, C.D., Fraumeni, J.F., Jr. The mortality experience of Army World War II chemical processing companies. *J. Occup. Med.* 23(Dec.):818–822, 1981.

Robinette, C.D. Re: Effects upon health of occupational exposure to microwave radiation RADAR (Letter to the Editor, Author's Reply). *Am. J. Epidemiol.* 113(Feb.):201–202, 1981.

Robinette, C.D. Methylated xanthines and pancreatic cancer (Letter to the Editor). *Lancet* 2(Oct.):754, 1981.

1982

Hrubec, Z., Neel, J.V. Contribution of familial factors to the occurrence of cancer before old age in twin veterans. *Am. J. Hum. Genet.* 34(July):658–671, 1982.

Norman, J.E., Jr. Breast cancer in women irradiated early in life. *Banbury Report* 11:433–450, 1982.

Shields, T.W., Higgins, G.A., Jr., Humphrey, E.W., Matthews, M.J., Keehn, R.J. Prolonged intermittent adjuvant chemotherapy with CCNU and hydroxyurea after resection of carcinoma of the lung. *Cancer* 50:1713–1721, 1982.

Shields, T.W., Higgins, G.A., Jr., Matthews, M.J., Keehn, R.J. Surgical resection in the management of small cell carcinoma of the lung. *J. Thorac. Cardiovasc. Surg.* 84(Oct.):481–488, 1982.

1983

Boice, J.D., Jr., Greene, M.H., Killen, J.Y., Jr., Ellenberg, S.S., Keehn, R.J., McFadden, E., Chen, T.T., Fraumeni, J.F. Leukemia and preleukemia after adjuvant treatment of gastrointestinal cancer with methyl-CCNU. *New Engl. J. Med.* 309(Nov.):1079–1084, 1983.

Higgins, G.A., Amadeo, J.H., Smith, D.E., Humphrey, E.W., Keehn, R.J. Efficacy of prolonged intermittent therapy with combined 5-FU and Me-CCNU following resection for gastric carcinoma: A Veterans Administration Surgical Oncology Group report. *Cancer* 52(Sept.):1105–1112, 1983.

Jablon, S. Characteristics of Current and Expected Dosimetry. Atomic bomb survivor data: Utilization and analysis. Pp. 143–152 in *Proceedings of a SIMS Conference*, Alta, Utah, September 12–16, 1983.

Jablon, S. Follow-up studies on A-bomb survivors: Implications for radiological protection. Pp. 167–180 in *Proceedings of the Health Physics Society*, Albuquerque, N.M., January 9–13, 1983. CONF-830101, 1983.

Jablon, S. Probability of Causation—Practical Problems. In J.J. Broerse, G.W. Bavendsen, H.B. Kal, and A.J. van der Kogel (eds.) *Proceedings of the 7th International Congress of Radiation Research*, July 3–8, 1983. The Netherlands: Martinus Nijhoff, 1983.

Kendler, K.S., Robinette, C.D. Month of birth by zygosity in the NAS–NRC Twin Registry. *Acta Genet. Med. Gemellol.* 32:113–116, 1983.

Kendler, K.S., Robinette, C.D. Schizophrenia in the NAS–NRC Twin Registry: A 16-year update. *Am. J. Psychiat.* 140(Dec.):1551–1563, 1983.

Norman, J.E., Jr., Cook, S.D., Dowling, P.C. Household pets among veterans with multiple sclerosis and age-matched controls. *Arch. Neurol.* 40:213–214, 1983.

Norman, J.E., Jr., Kurtzke, J.F., Beebe, G.W. Epidemiology of multiple sclerosis in U.S. veterans. 2: Latitude, climate, and the risk of multiple sclerosis. *J. Chron. Dis.* 36:551–559, 565–567, 1983.

1984

Higgins, G.A., Jr., Amadeo, J.H., McElhinney, J., McCaughan, J.J., Keehn, R.J. Efficacy of prolonged intermittent therapy with combined 5-fluorouracil and methyl-CCNU following resection for carcinoma of the large bowel: A Veterans Administration Surgical Oncology Group report. *Cancer* 53(Jan):1–8, 1984.

Higgins, G.A., Donaldson, R.C., Rogers, L.S., Juler, G.L., Keehn, R.J. Efficacy of MER immunotherapy when added to a regimen of 5-fluorouracil and methyl-CCNU following resection for carcinoma of the large bowel: A Veterans Administration Surgical Oncology Group report. *Cancer* 54(July):193–198, 1984.

Hrubec, Z., Robinette, C.D. The study of human twins in medical research. *New Engl. J. Med.* 310(Feb.):435–441, 1984.

Jablon, S. Epidemiologic perspectives in radiation carcinogenesis. Pp. 1–8 in J.D. Boice, Jr. and J.F. Fraumeni, Jr. (eds.) *Radiation Carcinogenesis: Epidemiology and Biological Significance, Progress in Cancer Research and Therapy*, Vol. 26. New York: Raven Press, 1984,

Matthews, K.A., Rosenman, R.H., Dembroski, T.M., Harris, E.L., MacDougall, J.M. Familial resemblance in components of the Type A behavior pattern: A reanalysis of the California Type A Twin Study. *Psychosomatic Medicine* 46:512–522, 1984.

1985

Campanale, R.P., Frey, C.F., Farias, R., Twomey, P.L., Guernsey, J.M., Keehn, R., Higgins, G. Reliability and sensitivity of frozen-section pancreatic biopsy. *Arch. Surg.* 120(Mar.):283–288, 1985.

Carmelli, D., Chesney, M.A., Ward, M.M., Rosenman, R.H. Twin similarity in cardiovascular stress response. *Health Psychology* 4:413–423, 1985.

Fabsitz, R., Feinleib, M., Hubert, H. Regression analysis of data with correlation errors: An example from the NHLBI twin study. *J. Chron. Dis.* 38:165–170, 1985.

Jablon, S. Atomic bomb survivors: Epidemiology and dose estimation. In *Epidemiology and Quantitation of Environmental Risk in Humans from Radiation and Other Agents*. New York: Plenum Press, 1985.

Jablon, S. The probability of causation: An approach to the problem of toxic torts, especially with respect to exposures to ionizing radiation. In *Epidemiology and Quantitation of Environmental Risk in Humans from Radiation and Other Agents*. New York: Plenum Press, 1985.

Jablon, S. Selection, follow-up and analysis in the Atomic Bomb Casualty Commission study. Presented at a Workshop on the Selection, Follow-up, and Analysis in Prospective Studies at the Waldorf Astoria Hotel, New York, October 3–5, 1983. *National Cancer Institute Monograph* 67:53–58, 1985.

Kendler, K.S. A twin study of individuals with both schizophrenia and alcoholism. *Br. J. of Psychiatry* 147:48–53, 1985.

Kurtzke, J.F., Beebe, G.W., Norman, J.E., Jr. Epidemiology of multiple sclerosis in U.S. veterans. III: Migration and the risk of MS. *Neurology* 35(5):672–678, 1985.

National Research Council, Committee on Toxicology. *Possible Long-Term Health Effects of Short-Term Exposure to Chemical Agents*, Vol. 3, *Final Report: Current Health Status of Test Subjects*. Washington, D.C: National Academy Press, 1985.

Robinette, C.D., Jablon, S., Preston, T.L. *Mortality of Nuclear Weapons Test Participants*. Medical Follow-up Agency, National Research Council. Washington, D.C.: National Academy Press, 1985.

1986

Higgins, G.A., Humphrey, E., Dwight, R.W., Roswit, B., Lee, L.E., Keehn, R.J. Preoperative radiation and surgery for cancer of the rectum. *Cancer* 58:352–359, 1986.

Kendler, K.S. A twin study of mortality in schizophrenia and neurosis. *Arch. Gen. Psychiatry.* 43(7):643–649, 1986.

Page, W.F. Prostate cancer (Letter to the Editor). *JNCI* 76(6):1259, 1986.

Reed, T. Blind assessment of zygosity using dermatoglyphics from the NHLBI Twin Study. *Amer. Dermatoglyphics Assoc. Newsletter* 5(3):6–11, 1986.

Spiritas, R., Beebe, G.W., Connelly, R.R., Wright, W.E., Peters, J.M., Sherwin, R.P., Henderson, B.E., Stark, A., Kovasznay, B.M., Davies, J.N.P., Vianna, N.J., Keehn, R.J., Ortega, L.G., Hochholzer, L., Wagner, J.C. Recent trends in mesothelioma incidence in the United States. *Am. J. of Indust. Med.* 9:397–407, 1986.

Stunkard, A.J., Foch, T.T., Hrubec, Z. A twin study of human obesity. *JAMA* 256(July):51–54, 1986.

1987

Carmelli, D., Rosenman, R.H., Chesney, M.A. Stability of the Type A structured interview and related questionnaires in a 10-year follow-up of an adult cohort of twins. *J. Behav. Med.* 10:513–525, 1987.

Christian, J.C., Borhani, N.O., Castelli, W.P., Fabsitz, R., Norton, J.A., Jr., Reed, T., Rosenman, R., Wood, P.D., Yu, P.L. Plasma cholesterol variation in the National Heart Lung and Blood Institute Twin Study. *Genet. Epidemiol.* 4:433–446, 1987.

Eisen, S., True, W., Goldberg, J., Henderson, W., Robinette, C.D. The Vietnam Era Twin (VET) Registry: Method of construction. *Acta Genet. Med. Gemellol.* 36:61–66, 1987.

Goldberg, J., True, W., Eisen, S., Henderson, W., Robinette, C.D. The Vietnam Era Twin (VET) Registry: Ascertainment bias. *Acta Genet. Med. Gemellol.* 36:67–78, 1987.

Jablon, S. Letter to the Editor: Response to Bross and Bross. *Am. J. Epid.* 126:1214, 1987.

Kalousdian, S., Fabsitz, R., Havlik, R., Christian, J., Roseman, R. Heritability of clinical chemistries in an older twin cohort: The NHLBI Twin Study. *Gen. Epidemiol.* 4:1–11, 1987.

Kendler, K.S., Tsuang, M.T., Hays, P. Age at onset in schizophrenia: A familial perspective. *Arch. of Gen. Psychiatry* 44(Oct.):881–890, 1987.

Luxenberg, J.S., May, C., Haxby, J.V., Grady, C., Moore, S., Berg, G., White, B. J., Robinette, C.D., Rapoport, S.I. Cerebral metabolism, anatomy, and cognition in monozygotic twins discordant for dementia of the Alzheimer type. *J. Neurol. Neurosurg. Psy.* 50(3):333–340, 1987.

Newman, B., Selby, J.V., King, M.C., Slemenda, C., Fabsitz, R., Friedman, G.D. Concordance for type 2 (non-insulin-dependent) diabetes mellitus in male twins. *Diabetologia* 30:764–768, 1987.

Page, W.F. Migration biases in address tracing by commercial firms. *Am. J. Epid.* 125:163–165, 1987.

Page, W.F. Mortality and morbidity selection effects among U.S. veterans. *J. Occup. Med.* 29(12):975–978, 1987.

Seeff, L.B., Beebe, G.W., Hoofnagle, J.H., Norman, J.E., Buskell-Bales, Z., Waggoner, J.G., Kaplowitz, N., Koff, R.S., Petrini, J.L., Jr., Schiff, E.R., Shorey, J., Stanley, M.M. A serologic follow-up of the 1942 epidemic of post-vaccinal hepatitis in the United States Army. *N. Engl. J. Med.* 316(16):965–970, 1987.

1988

Carmelli, D., Rosenman, R., Chesney, M., Fabsitz, R., Lee, M., Borhani, N. Genetic heritability and shared environmental influences of Type A measures in the NHLBI Twin Study. *Am. J. Epidemiol.* 127:1041–1052, 1988.

Carmelli, D., Rosenman, R.H., Swan, G.E. The Cook and Medley HO Scale: A heritability analysis in adult male twins. *Psychosomatic Medicine* 50:165–174, 1988.

Fabsitz, R.R., Kalousdian, S., Carmelli, D., Robinette, D., Christian, J.C. Characteristics of participants and nonparticipants in the NHLBI Twin Study. *Acta Genet. Med. Gemellol.* 37:217–228, 1988.

Jablon, S. *How to be Quantitative About Radiation Risk Estimates.* Lecture No.11, The Lauriston S. Taylor Lecture Series in Radiation Protection and Measurements, Bethesda, Md.: NCRP, 1988.

Swan, G.E., Carmelli, D., Rosenman, R.H. Psychological characteristics in twins discordant for smoking behavior: A matched-twin-pair analysis. *Addict. Behav.* 13:51–60, 1988.

1989

Bogle, A.C. A study of A-B ridge count asymmetry as a marker of developmental canalization. Ph.D. thesis. Indiana University, 1989.

Centerwall, B.S., Robinette, C.D. Twin concordance for dishonorable discharge from the military: With a review of the genetics of antisocial behaviour. *Compr. Psychiatry* 30:442–446, 1989.

Christian, J.C., You, P.L., Slemenda, C.W., Johnston, C.C., Jr. Heritability of bone mass: A longitudinal study in aging male twins. *Am. J. Hum. Genet* 44:429–433, 1989.

Fabsitz, R.R., Nam, J., Gart, J., Stunkard, A., Price, R.A., Wilson, P.W.F. HLA associations with obesity. Hum. Heredity 39:156–164, 1989.

McLaughlin, J.K., Hrubec, Z., Linet, M.S., Heineman, E.F., Blot, W.J., Fraumeni, J.F. Cigarette smoking and leukemia (Letter). *JNCI* 81(16) (Aug.):1262–1263, 1989.

Selby, J.V., Newman, B., Fabsitz, R.R., King, M.C., Friedman, G.D. Evidence of genetic influence on central body fat in middle-aged twins. *Hum. Biol.* 61(2):179–193, 1989.

1990

Breitner, J.C., Murphy, E.A., Folstein, M.F., Magruder-Habib, K. Twin studies of Alzheimer's disease: An approach to etiology and prevention. *Neurobiol. Aging* 1:641–648, 1990.

Breitner, J.C.S.,Welsh, K.A., Magruder-Habib, K.M., Churchill, C.M., Robinette C.D., Folstein, M.F., Murphy, E.A., Priolo, C.C., Brandt, J. Alzheimer's disease in the NAS Registry of aging twin veterans. 1: Pilot investigations. *Dementia* 1:297–303, 1990.

Carmelli, D., Swan, G.E., Robinette, D., Fabsitz, R.R. Heritability of substance use in the NAS–NRC Twin Registry. *Acta Genet. Med. Gemellol.* 39:91–98, 1990.

Carmelli, D., Swan, G.E., Rosenman, R.H. The heritability of the Cook and Medley Hostility Scale revisited. *J. Soc. Behav.* 5:263–276, 1990.

Carmelli, D., Swan, G.E., Rosenman, R.H. Self-ratings and perceptions of Type A traits in adult twins. *J. Soc. Behav.* 5:263–276, 1990.

Christian, J.C., Carmelli, D., Castelli, W.P., Fabsitz, R.R., Grim, C.E., Meaney, F.J., Norton, J.A., Jr., Reed, T., Williams, C.J., Wood, P.J. High density lipoprotein cholesterol: A sixteen year longitudinal study in aging male twins. *Arteriosclerosis* 10:1020–1025, 1990.

Havlik, R.J., Fabsitz, R.R., Kalousdian, S., Borhani, N.O., Christian, J.C. Dietary protein and blood pressure in monozygotic twins. *Prev. Med.* 19:31–39, 1990.

Newman, B., Selby, J.V., Quesenberry, C.P., Jr., King, M.C., Friedman, G.D., Fabsitz, R.R. Nongenetic influences of obesity on other cardiovascular disease risk factors: An analysis of identical twins. *Am. J. Public Health* 80:675–678, 1990.

Page, W.F., Norman, J.E., Hrubec, Z. Colon cancer mortality among amputees. *JNCI* 82(2):154–155, 1990.

Reed, T., Fabsitz, R.R., Quiroga, J. Family history of heart disease with respect to mean twin-pair cholesterol and subsequent ischemic heart disease in the NHLBI Twin Study. *Genet. Epidemiol.* 7:335–347, 1990.

Selby, J.V., Newman, B., Quesenberry, C.P., Jr., Fabsitz, R.R., Carmelli, D., Meaney, F.J., Slemenda, C. Genetics and behavioral influences on body fat distribution. *Int. J. Obes.* 14:593–602, 1990.

Swan, G.E., Carmelli, D., Reed, T., Harshfield, G.A., Fabsitz, R.R., Eslinger, P.J. Heritability of cognitive function in aging twins: The NHLBI Twin Study. *Arch. Neurol.* 47:259–262, 1990.

Swan, G.E., Carmelli, D., Rosenman, R.H. Cook and Medley hostility and the Type A behavior pattern: Psychological correlates of two coronary-prone behaviors. *J. Soc. Behav.* 5:89–106, 1990.

Swan, G.E., Carmelli, D., Rosenman, R.H. Psychological correlates of two measures of coronary-prone hostility. *Psychosomatics* 30:270–278, 1990.

Swan, G.E., Carmelli, R.H., Rosenman, D., Fabsitz, R.R., Christian, J.C. Smoking and alcohol consumption in adult male twins: Genetic heritability and shared environmental influences. *J. Subst. Abuse* 2(1):39–50, 1990.

1991

Carmelli, D., Swan, G.E., Robinette, D. Substance Use in World War II Veteran Twins: A Genetic Analysis. Pp. 19–34. in W.F. Page (ed.) *Epidemiology in Military and Veteran Populations*. Washington, D.C.: National Academy Press, 1991.

Carmelli, D., Ward, M.M., Reed, T., Grim, C.E., Harshfield, G.A., Fabsitz, R.R. Genetic effects on cardiovascular responses to cold and mental activity in late adulthood. *Am. I. Hyperten.* 4:239–244, 1991.

Elashoff, J.D., Cantor, R.M., Shain, S. Power and validity of methods to identify variability genes. *Genet. Epidemiol.* 8:381–388, 1991.

Engdahl, B.E., Page, W.F. Pyschological Effects of Military Captivity. Pp. 49–66 in W.F. Page (ed.) *Epidemiology in Military and Veteran Populations*. Washington, D.C.: National Academy Press, 1991.

Engdahl, B.E., Page, W.F., Miller, T.W. Age, education, maltreatment, and social support as predictors of chronic depression in former prisoners of War. *Soc. Psychiatry Psychiatr. Epidemiol.* 26:63–67, 1991.

Kumar, A., Schapiro, M.B., Grady, C.L., Matocha, M.F., Haxby, J.V., Moore, A.M., Luxenbert, J.S., St. Goerge-Hyslop, P.H., Robinette, C.D., Ball, M.J., Rapoport, S. Atomic, metabolic, neuropsychological, and molecular genetic studies of three pairs of identical twins discordant for dementia of the Alzheimer's type. *Arch. Neurol.* 48:160–168, 1991.

Lamon-Fava, S., Jimenez, D., Christian, J.C., Fabsitz, R.R., Carmelli, D., Castelli, W.P., Ordovas, J.M., Wilson, P.W., Schaefer, E.J. Heritability of apolipoprotein A-I, B, and low-density lipoprotein subclasses and concordances for lipoprotein. (a). *Atherosclerosis* 91(1–2):97–106, 1991.

Page, W.F. *Epidemiology in Military and Veteran Populations: Proceedings of the Second Biennial Conference*, March 7, 1990. Washington, D.C.: National Academy Press, 1991.

Page, W.F. Using longitudinal data to estimate nonresponse bias. *Soc. Psychiatry Psychiatr. Epidemiol.* 26:127–131, 1991.

Page, W.F., Engdahl, B.E. Age, education, maltreatment, and social support as predictors of chronic depression in former prisoners of war. *Soc. Psychiatry and Psychiatr. Epidemiol.* 26:63–67, 1991.

Page, W.F., Engdahl, B.E., Eberly, R.E. Prevalence and correlates of depressive symptoms among former prisoners of war. *J. Nerv. Ment. Dis.* 179:670–677, 1991.

Reed, T., Carmelli, D., Rosenman, R.H. Effects of placentation on selected Type A behaviors in adult males in the National Heart, Lung, and Blood Institute (NHLBI) Twin Study. *Behav. Genet.* 21:9–19, 1991.

Reed, T., Fabsitz, R.R., Selby, J.V., Carmelli, D. Genetic influences and grip strength norms in the National Heart, Lung, and Blood Institute Twin Study males aged 59–69. *Ann. Hum. Biol.* 18(5) 425–432, 1991.

Reed, T., Christian, J.C., Wood, P.D., Schaefer, E.J. Influence of placentation on high density lipoproteins in adult males: The NHLBI Twin Study. *Acta Genet. Med. Gemollol.* 40:353–359, 1991.

Reed, T., Malinow, M.R., Christian, J.C., Upson, B. Estimates of heritability for plasma homocyst(e)ine levels in aging adult male twins. *Clin. Genet.* 39:425–428, 1991.

Reed, T., Quiroga, J., Selby, J.V., Carmelli, D., Christian, J.C., Fabsitz, R.R., Grim, C.E. Concordance of ischemic heart disease in the National Heart, Lung, and Blood Institute Twin Study after 14–18 years of follow-up. *J. of Clin. Epidemiol.* 44(8):797–805, 1991.

Ron, E., Gridley, G., Hrubec, Z., Page, W.F., Arora, S., Fraumeni, J.F. Acromegaly and gastrointestinal cancer. *Cancer* 68:1673–1677, 1991.

Roy, A., Segal, N.L., Centerwal, B.S., Robinette, C.D. Suicide in twins. *Arch. Gen. Psychiatry* 48:29–32, 1991.

Selby, J.V., Newman, B., Quiroga, J., Christian, J.C., Austin, M.A., Fabsitz, R.R. Concordance for dyslipidemic hypertension in male twins. *JAMA* 265:2079–2084, 1991.

Selby, J.V., Reed, T., Newman, B., Fabsitz, R.R., Carmelli, D. Effects of selective return on estimates of heritability for body mass index in the National Heart, Lung, and Blood Institute Twin Study. *Genet. Epidemiol.* 8(6):371–380, 1991.

1992

Brass, L.M., Isaacsohn, J.L., Merikangas, K.R., Robinette, C.D. A study of twins and stroke. *Stroke* 23(2):1–3, 1992.

Breitner, J.C.S., Murphy, E.A. Twin studies of Alzheimer's disease. II: Some predictions under a genetic model. *Am. J. Med. Genet.* 44:628–634, 1992.

Carmelli, D., Swan, G.E., Robinette, C.D., Fabsitz, R.R. Genetic influence on smoking: A study of male twins. *N. Engl. J. Med.* 327(12):829–833, 1992.

Fabsitz, R.R., Carmelli, D., Hewitt, J.K. Evidence for independent genetic influences on obesity in middle age. *Int. J. Obes.* 16:657–666, 1992.

Kurtzke, J.F., Page, W.F., Murphy, F.M., Norman, J.E. Epidemiology of multiple sclerosis in U.S. veterans. IV: Age at onset. *Neuroepidemiology* 11:226–235, 1992.

Murphy, E.A., Breitner, J.C.S. Threshold model in the genetics of age-dependent disease in twins. 1: General principles as applied to Alzheimer's disease. *Am. J. Med. Genet.* 42:842–850, 1992.

Page, W.F. *The Health of Former Prisoners of War—Results From the Medical Examination Survey of Former POWs of World War II and the Korean Conflict.* Washington, D.C.: National Academy Press, 1992.

Page, W.F. VA mortality reporting for World War II Army veterans, (Letter to the Editor). *Am. J. Public Health* 82(1):124–125, 1992.

Seeff, L.B., Buskell-Bales, Z., Wright, E.C., Durako, S.J., Alter, H.J. The long-term mortality of transfusion-associated non-A, non-B hepatitis in the United States. *N. Engl. J. Med.* 327(27):1906–1911, 1992.

Slemenda, C.W., Christian, J.C., Reed, T., Reister, T.K., Williams, C.J., Johnson, C.C., Jr. Long-term bone loss in men: Effects of genetic and environmental factors. *Ann. Int. Med.* 117:286–291, 1992.

Swan, G.E., LaRue, A., Carmelli, D., Reed, T., Fabsitz, R.R. Decline in cognitive performance in aging twins: Heritability and biobehavioral predictors from the National Heart, Lung, and Blood Institute Twin Study. *Arch. Neurol.* 49(5) 476–481, 1992.

Terry, R.B., Page, W.F., Haskell, W.L. Waist/hip ratio, body mass index and premature cardiovascular disease mortality in U.S. Army veterans during a twenty-three year follow-up study. *Int. J. Obes.* 16:417–423, 1992.

1993

Brandt, J., Welsh, K.A., Breitner, J.C.S., Folstein, M.F., Helms, M., Christian, J.C. Hereditary influences on cognitive functioning in older men. A study of 4000 twin pairs. *Arch. Neurol.* 50(6):599–603, 1993.

Carmelli, D., Heath, A.C., Robinette, D. Genetic analysis of drinking behavior in World War II veteran twins. *Genet. Epidemiol.* 10:201–213, 1993.

Carmelli, D., Swan, G.E., Robinette, D. The relationship between quitting smoking and changes in drinking in World War II veteran twins. *J. Subst. Abuse* 5:103–116, 1993.

Colletto, G.M., Cardon, L.R., Fulker, D.W. A genetic and environmental time series analysis of blood pressure in male twins. *Genet. Epidemiol.* 10:533–538, 1993.

Dunlap, N.E., Ballinger, S., Reed, T., Christian, J.C., Koopman, W.J., Briles, D.E. The use of monozygotic and dizygotic twins to estimate the effects of inheritance on the levels of immunoglobulin isotypes and antibodies to phosphocholine. *Clin. Immunol. Immunopathol.* 66(2):176–180, 1993.

Engdahl, B.E., Harkness, A.R., Eberly, R.E., Page, W.F., Bielinski, J. Structural models of captivity trauma, resilience, and trauma response among former prisoners of war 20 to 40 years after release. *Soc. Psychiatry and Psychiatr. Epidemiol.* 28:109–115, 1993.

Grove, J.S., Zhao, L.P., Quiaolt, F. Correlation analysis of twin data with repeated measures based on generalized estimating equations. *Genet. Epidemiol.* 10:539–544, 1993.

Narkun-Burgess, D.M., Nolan, C.R., Norman, J.E., Page, W.F., Miller, P.L., Meyer, T.W. Forty-five year follow-up after uninephrectomy. *Kidney Int.* 43:1110–1115, 1993.

Norman, J.E., Beebe, G.W., Hoofnagle, J.H., Seef, L.B. Mortality follow-up of the 1942 epidemic of hepatitis B in the U.S. Army. *Hepatology* 18(4):790–797, 1993.

Page, W.F., Kurtzke, J.F., Murphy, F.M., Norman, J.E. Epidemiology of multiple sclerosis in U.S. veterans. V: Ancestry and the risk of multiple sclerosis. *Ann. Neurol.* 33:632–639, 1993.

Page, W.F., Norman, J.E., Benenson, A.S. Long term follow-up of Army recruits immunized with adjuvant influenza vaccine. *Vaccine Research* 3(2):141–149, 1993.

Reed, T., Carmelli, D., Selby, J.V., Fabsitz, R.R. The NHLBI Male Veteran Twin Study data. *Genet. Epidemiol.* 10:513–517, 1993.

Schwartz, J.E., Yuan, H., Mendell, N.R., Finch, S.J. LISREL modeling of high density lipoprotein cholesterol (HDL) levels in male twins. *Genet. Epidemiol.* 10:545–549, 1993.

Williams, C., Wijesiri, U.W.L. Lipid data from NHLBI veteran twins: Interpreting genetic analyses when model assumptions fail. *Genet. Epidemiol.* 10: 551–556, 1993.

1994

Breitner, J.C.S., Gau, B.A., Welsh, K.A., Plasman, B.L., McDonald, W.M., Helms, M.J., Anthony, J.C. Inverse association of anti-inflammatory treatments and Alzheimer's disease. *Neurology* 44(2):227–232, 1994.

Breitner, J.C.S., Welsh, K.A., Robinette, C.D., Gau, B.A., Folstein, M.F., Brandt, J. Alzheimer's disease in the NAS–NRC Registry of aging twins. II: Longitudinal findings in a pilot series. *Dementia* 5(2):99–105, 1994.

Braun, M.M., Caporaso, N.E., Page, W.F., Hoover, R.N. Genetic component of lung cancer: Cohort study of twins. *Lancet* 344:440–443, 1994.

Braun, M.M., Caporaso, N.E., Brinton, L., Page, W.F. Re: Twin membership and breast cancer risk (Letter). *Am. J. Epidemiol.* 140(6):575–576, 1994.

Braun, M.M., Haupt, R., Caporaso, N.E. The National Academy of Sciences–National Research Council veteran twin registry. *Acta Genet. Med. Gemellol.* 43:89–94, 1994.

Cardon, L.R., Carmelli, D., Fabsitz, R.R., Reed, T. Genetic and environmental correlations between obesity and body fat distribution in adult male twins. *Hum. Biol.* 66(3):465–479, 1994.

Carmelli, D., Cardon, L.R., Fabsitz, R. Clustering of hypertension, diabetes, and obesity in adult male twins: Same genes or same environment? *Am. J. Hum. Genet.* 55:566–573, 1994.

Carmelli, D., Robinette, C.D., Fabsitz, R. Concordance, discordance and prevalence of hypertension in World War II male veteran twins. *J. Hypertens.* 12(3):323–328, 1994.

Carmelli, D., Selby, J.V., Quiroga, J., Reed, T., Fabsitz, R.R., Christian, J.C. 16-year incidence of ischemic heart disease in the NHLBI twin study: A classification of subjects into high- and low-risk groups. *Ann. Epidemiol.* 4(3):198–204, 1994.

Fabsitz, R.R., Sholinsky, P., Carmelli, D. Genetic influences on adult weight gain and maximum body mass index in male twins. *Am. J. Epidemiol.* 140(8):711–720, 1994.

Gridley, G., Klippel, J.H., Hoover, R.N., Fraumeni, J.F. Incidence of cancer among men with felty syndrome. *Ann. Intern. Med.* 1120(1):35–39, 1994.

Jarvik, G.P., Austin, M.A., Fabsitz, R.R., Auwerx, J., Reed, T., Christian, J.C., Deeb, S. Genetic influences on age-related change in total cholesterol, low density lipoprotein cholesterol, and triglyceride levels: longitudinal apolipoprotein E genotype effects. *Genet. Epidemiol.* 11:375–384, 1994.

Page, W.F. NAS–NRC Twin Registry 1995 Survey (Letter). *Am. J. Hum. Genet.* 52:254, 1994.

Page, W.F., Engdahl, B.E. A tradition of VA-supported research on POWs. *VA Practitioner* 11(6):49–54, 1994.

Page, W.F., Ostfeld, A.M. Malnutrition and subsequent ischemic heart disease in former prisoners of war of World War II and the Korean conflict. *J. Clin. Epidemiol.* 147(12):1437–1441, 1994.

Partin, A.W., Page, W.F., Lee, B.R., Sanda, M.G., Miller, R.N., Walsh, P.C. Concordance rates for benign prostatic disease among twins suggest hereditary influence. *Urology* 44(5):646–650, 1994.

Reed, T., Carmelli, D., Swan, G.E., Breitner, J.C.S., Welsh, K.A., Jarvik, G.P., Deeb, S., Auwerx, J. Lower cognitive performance in normal older adult male twins carrying the apolipoprotein E e4 allele. *Arch. Neurol.* 51:1189–1192, 1994.

Reed, T., Slemenda, C.W., Viken, R.J., Christian, J.C., Carmelli, D., Fabsitz, R.R. Correlations of alcohol consumption with related covariates and heritability estimates in older adult males over a 14- to 18-year period: The NHLBI Twin Study. *Alcohol Clin. Exp. Res.* 18(3):702–710, 1994.

Reed, T., Tracy, R.P., Fabsitz, R.R. Minimal genetic influences on plasma fibrinogen level in adult males in the NHLBI Twin Study. *Clin. Genet.* 45(2): 71–77, 1994.

1995

Breitner, J.C.S., Welsh, K.A., Gau, B.A., McDonald, W.M., Steffens, D.C., Saunders, A.M., Magruder, K.M., Helms, M.S., Plassman, B.L., Folstein, M.F., Brandt, J., Robinette, C.D., Page, W.F. Alzheimer's disease in the National Academy of Sciences–National Research Council Registry of aging twin veterans. *Arch. Neurol.* 52(Aug.), 1995.

Braun, M.M., Caporaso, N.E., Page, W.F., Hoover, R.N. A cohort study of twins and cancer. *Cancer Epidemiol. Biomarkers Prev.* 4:469–473, 1995.

Braun, M.M., Caporaso, N.E., Page, W.F., Hoover, R.N. Prevalence of a history of testicular cancer in a cohort of elderly twins. *Acta Genet. Med. Gemellol.* 44:189–192, 1995.

Carmelli, D., Swan, G.E., Page, W.F., Christian, J.C. World War II veteran male twins who are discordant for alcohol consumption: 24-year mortality. *Am. J. Public Health* 85:99–101, 1995.

Christian, J.C., Reed, T., Carmelli, D., Page, W.F., Norton, J.A., Breitner, J.C.S. Self-reported alcohol intake and cognition in aging twins. *J. Stud. Alcohol* 56:414–416, 1995.

National Research Council. *Adverse Reproductive Outcomes in Families of Atomic Veterans: The Feasibility of Epidemiology Studies.* Washington, D.C.: National Academy Press, 1995.

National Research Council. *Health Consequences of Service During the Persian Gulf War: Initial Findings and Recommendations for Immediate Action.* Washington, D.C.: National Academy Press, 1995.

Non-small Cell Lung Cancer Collaborative Group. Chemotherapy in non-small cell lung cancer: A meta-analysis using updated data on individual patients from 52 randomised clinical trials. *Br. Med. J.* 311:899–909, 1995.

Page, W.F. Annotation: The National Academy of Sciences, National Research Council Twin Registry. *Am. J. Public Health* 85:617–618, 1995.

Page, W.F., Braun, M.M., Caporaso, N.E. Ascertainment of mortality in U.S. veteran population: World War II veteran twins. *Mil. Med.* 160(7):351, 1995.

Page, W.F., Mack, T.M., Kurtzke, J.F., Murphy, F.M., Norman, J.E. Epidemiology of multiple sclerosis in U.S. veterans. 6: Population ancestry and surname ethnicity as risk factors for multiple sclerosis. *Neuroepidemiology* 14:286–296, 1995.

Plassman, B.L., Welsh, K.A., Helms, M., Brandt, J., Page, W.F., Breitner, J.C.S. Intelligence and education as predictors of cognitive state in late life: A 50-year follow-up. *Neurology* 45:1446–1450, 1995.

1996

Brass, L.M., Hartigan, P.M., Page, W.F., Concato, J. Importance of cerebrovascular disease in studies of myocardial infarction. *Stroke* 27:1173–1176, 1996.

Carmelli, D., Swan, G.E., Page, W.F. 24-years of mortality in smoking-discordant U.S. male veteran twins. *Int. J. Epidemiol.* 25:554–559, 1996.

Johnson, J.C., Thaul, S., Page, W.F., Crawford, H. *Mortality of Veteran Participants in the Crossroads Nuclear Test.* Washington, D.C.: National Academy Press, 1996.

National Research Council. *Health Consequences of Service During the Persian Gulf War: Recommendations for Research and Information Systems.* Washington, D.C.: National Academy Press, 1996.

Page, W.F., Mahan, C.M., Kang, H.K. Vital status ascertainment through the files of the Department of Veterans Affairs and the Social Security Administration. *Ann. Epidemiol.* 6(2):102–109, 1996.

Petersdorf, R.G., Page, W.F., Thaul, S. *The Interactions of Drugs, Biologics, and Chemicals in U.S. Military Forces.* Washington, D.C.: National Academy Press, 1996.

Index

About the Authors

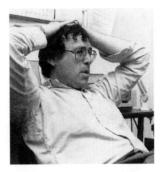

Edward D. Berkowitz, Ph.D., is a professor of history at the George Washington University. He has written widely on history and social welfare policy, including *To Improve Human Health: A History of the Institute of Medicine,* which was published in 1998.

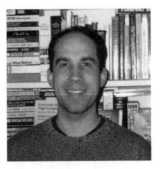

Mark J. Santangelo is a Ph.D. candidate in history at the George Washington University, specializing in twentieth-century American history. He served as chief researcher for *To Improve Human Health: A History of the Institute of Medicine.*